Rachel McGrath grew up in Redcliffe, a seaside town in Queensland, Australia, where she studied Business, before moving to the United Kingdom in her early thirties. She currently lives just north of London, where she met and married her husband. She has a professional career in human resources. Rachel has always had a passion for writing both fiction and non-fiction, creating many short stories from her early teens as well as smaller pieces of work that have never been published.

Embracing the Storm is the sequel to Rachel's first published novel, a memoir capturing a difficult time in her life; she is passionate about sharing this with a wider audience.

Rachel has since published several other books, including Children's fiction stories. She has received acclaim through various book prizes for both her non-fiction and fiction publications.

Rachel has a built strong, world-wide following via her personal blog www.findingthrainbow.net

Rachel McGrath

Embracing the Storm

McGRATH HOUSE PAPERBACK

© Copyright 2017
Rachel McGrath

The right of Rachel McGrath to be identified as author of this work has been asserted by her in accordance with the Copyright, Designs and Patents Act 1988.

All Rights Reserved
No reproduction, copy or transmission of this publication may be made without written permission.
No paragraph of this publication may be reproduced, copied or transmitted save with the written permission of the publisher, or in accordance with the provisions of the Copyright Act 1956 (as amended).

Any person who commits any unauthorised act in relation to this publication may be liable to criminal prosecution and civil claims for damages.

Although the author and publisher have made every effort to ensure that the information in this book was correct at press time, the author and publisher do not assume and hereby disclaim any liability to any party for any loss, damage, or disruption caused by errors or omissions, whether such errors or omissions result from negligence, accident, or any other cause.

ISBN 978- 1542558952

First Edition 2017 by McGrath House

This book is dedicated to my family and friends who have been with me through this journey.

My husband, who is my soul mate and he has been my rock through some incredibly difficult times on our journey to become parents. Thank you for always encouraging me to chase my dreams, and for never giving up with me.

My mother, who has been an empathetic ear when I've needed it, as well as my proof-reader and sanity check for the very first version of this manuscript.

My father, who is fighting an even greater battle right now, but always does so with a smile and a positive outlook.

Finding the Rainbow

I have not yet met one woman who expected to face any obstacles with their own fertility after deciding to start a family. The women I have met via my blog or in person, all told me that they were taken by surprise. They didn't anticipate that their journey to become parents would be so hard, or even impossible.

Perhaps you have read my earlier memoir, *Finding the Rainbow*, or perhaps not. I can assure you that this second story of mine requires no pre-requisite reading. *Finding the Rainbow*, in its shortest version, was the story that led to me finding out that I would struggle with conceiving and carrying a baby to full term. I said it then, and I'll say it now, I never thought getting pregnant or staying pregnant would be so difficult.

Finding the Rainbow didn't end with the baby we had wished for, but it did end with the hope of a family someday in our future. In reality, not all stories have the happy ending we hope for or expect. Nonetheless, I have been overwhelmed by the response and feedback from my first memoir. That's why I knew I couldn't leave my story there; I had to write the second chapter to my journey.

Before we start, I will remind my readers that this is a memoir, not a fairy-tale. In writing this next story I wanted to remain transparent and honest about my experiences, my feelings and my thoughts. Fighting the battle against my infertility and my body has led to some of the toughest moments I have ever encountered in my life, both mentally and physically. I write this story with all of my heart and soul.

As a woman who has now had four early pregnancy losses and no healthy baby to date, my story is sadly one that many couples face daily. *Finding the Rainbow* describes my struggles to conceive, despite believing that a family would come easily to us as a couple. I was fit and healthy, and I had no obvious 'female' issues. Yet Mother Nature was not cooperating with my desire to become a mother. Having a baby should have been one of the most natural experiences. However, the reality is that infertility affects as many as one in four women. With my age thrown into the mix, the odds were against us. Facing the obstacles I did, as well as the loss, the frustration, and the not knowing of why this was happening – that was my story.

I was married at thirty-five, which is not unusual these days. In fact, most of my friends have married in their mid to late thirties. So, when it came to family planning, we had very exact plans. We decided to wait exactly twelve months after our wedding before considering children. We wanted to enjoy a year of marriage and believed our first pregnancy would happen very quickly and easily. We were wrong.

As a couple, we never expected infertility to happen to us. But then again, nobody does. It was all an entirely new world to me, and I was quite unprepared for the physical and emotional rollercoaster that was involved. I hadn't really thought about it before, but soon I became one of those fertility statistics you hear about. Given my age, I should have perhaps been a little more aware – but I wasn't. We were encouraged to try again, and at the time after our first loss, we thought naively that our bad luck would pass. It didn't.

All four of my pregnancies ended within the first trimester, and each one was equally heart-breaking, but on their own different and challenging. I look back now and I know I was lucky to even fall pregnant as I realise many women struggle to reach that first hurdle. In retrospect, I will always retain the dates of each of those pregnancies, and those little angel babies I would never meet. It still hurts my heart to think about those times, and I deeply feel for any woman who has to experience what I did, even once. It's cruel and it's heartbreaking; it's a promise of hope that is suddenly ripped away.

It all started to feel as though I was playing a game of odds, and I was constantly reminded that I was a statistic on the fertility charts. I am the one in four who have experienced early pregnancy loss. I'm also in the one percent of women who've sadly lost three or more pregnancies in a row. Being in my late thirties, I was told that the odds of pregnancy loss were becoming greater with time, and that any baby we did have had a high probability of being born with a disability or impairment.

Still, I approached our dreams of having a baby with optimism. Once we fell pregnant that first time, we didn't seem to have a problem conceiving. In fact, we fell pregnant four times in under two years. The problem was that I couldn't carry the baby past the first trimester. Each pregnancy ended with the devastating news that the baby had stopped growing and there was no heartbeat. After four miscarriages, I felt lost, frustrated and cheated by my own body. Yet I still had to hold onto the belief that we would one day be blessed with a child of our own.

Throughout it all, I discovered that the topic of infertility and miscarriage was often hushed or deemed uncomfortable to discuss openly. Many couples don't share the challenges they face on their road to parenthood, and there seemed to be an unspoken agreement that it is not 'right' to discuss your pregnancy until you successfully reach the first trimester. For me, personally, I struggled with keeping quiet. In a time of expected silence and secrecy, I needed the people around me to keep me positive and sometimes sane. I needed support and help to get me through my fears and the anxiety I was facing. Having faced the loss of miscarriage, I had a constant and uncontrollable fear of losing another baby from that very first positive pregnancy test, and with each miscarriage that anxiety grew even stronger.

With each loss, my husband and I went from elation to devastation, and each time it happened, the hopelessness of our situation started to grow. When we lost our last baby, we followed a number of steps to investigate the matter seriously. I had a D&C (dilation and curettage) procedure to analyse the foetus, and underwent various blood tests to look at any other factors that may be causing our early losses.

Whilst no obvious concerns were found with the tissue they collected from the D&C, I was advised that I had 'sticky blood' or protein S deficiency. What that meant was that I had a possible solution; perhaps it was my blood that had caused these early losses. The specialists predicted that perhaps my blood was too thick or it was clotting in those very early weeks. With a small foetus measuring only one or two millimetres as its heart first starts to pump blood, this prognosis seemed to make sense. My blood thickening and clotting was causing growth issues. The poor little heart couldn't get enough blood flow and ultimately it would stop beating. Suddenly, all hope was not lost, and our specialist advised us that the solution could be as simple as blood thinning injections throughout my next pregnancy.

After almost three years of feeling as though we were on a continuous cycle leading nowhere, we could suddenly move forward, with some hope that our next pregnancy may finally provide us with our much longed for rainbow baby.

We had travelled through this devastating storm, and it had left its damage on both my husband and me, emotionally and physically. It was the promise of the rainbow when the thunder and rain stopped and the clouds subsided that kept us going through all that pain. The damage from the storm is never really forgotten, but it's the promise of that colourful rainbow that always gave us hope and courage to keep moving forward. It was our pursuit of our rainbow baby that drove our persistence, and finally we could see the light at the end of the storm.

Whilst we have not yet conquered the dark clouds, I'm prepared to face the torment and the rain head on. We will embrace this storm wholeheartedly, facing our hopes, fears and anxieties for a new beginning tomorrow.

This is the next chapter in our story…

Forecasting the Odds

After experiencing four unexplained losses and now reaching my third year of trying to conceive, I was becoming a little philosophical. My first baby would now be a toddler; our lives could have been so very different today.

Nevertheless, the room we planned to turn into a nursery remains empty, and in fact we are not really sure what to do with it right now. Life just keeps moving forward. Around us, our friends and family have toddlers and babies, and we continue to be branded as the 'carefree couple without kids'. We joke about it amongst others, that we have no responsibilities and can focus on our careers, but deep down there is always something missing.

Despite the setbacks, I am still on this treadmill of 'trying to conceive', and whilst at times I feel out of breath and exhausted I'm determined to keep going. Finding out that I had a diagnosis gave me that extra push to run faster. It is actually quite sad how excited I felt when I found out that I had 'sticky blood'. At least it felt as though there was a way forward, and to me it all made complete sense. Each of my pregnancies had never progressed past seven weeks, two of them had no heartbeat, and with the other two, the heartbeat was slow, before stopping altogether. Those tiny little foetuses were never able to get a proper blood flow to grow and develop. For me, the solution was now straightforward and doable. A simple daily blood thinning injection was all I needed before and throughout my future pregnancies. The results were proven to help women like me carry a baby to full term. My hope was back!

We were ready and waiting to start again. It had been almost two months since our D&C when the results were confirmed, so essentially we were ready to go. I just needed my cycle to return to normal.

After my previous miscarriages, it had taken sometimes around two months for my cycle to return. Now, I will openly admit that I'm not the most patient person in the world, and the anxiety of waiting for a period to arrive when you have nothing to go by is frustrating, to say the least. I had been lucky, with a regular twenty-eight day cycle each month, but I needed that cycle so I could waste no more time and get pregnant again.

By the third month I was becoming a little anxious. Still nothing, and, in fact, I was sure that I was feeling period pain every few weeks, but there was nothing to show for it. I found myself constantly running to the toilet to check, hoping to see any sign at all. I went to my local doctor who assured me that due to the D&C it could just be taking a little longer to rectify. As I hit the fourth month with no cycle, I returned to my doctor, insisting that I should be referred to a specialist. I knew I was feeling my period cycle each month, but my body wasn't physically cooperating. Something was wrong.

I had several investigative scans, and it was found that my uterine lining was not thickening. It was all a learning curve for me. As a part of the female cycle the lining has to thicken in readiness for ovulation and implantation. The fact that mine wasn't thickening meant that something wasn't quite working. I was given a series of medications to try to kick-start my cycle over the next two months, and yet still nothing. I could tell my body wanted to menstruate as I could feel the pains that came with each period, but nothing happened. It was now over six months on, and I was completely frustrated. Again another hurdle I had to face on this stormy road. I was ready to go, but my body wasn't even letting me start!

I felt a growing anxiety as I continued to explore options with different specialists, all telling me that eventually my body would rectify this problem. Yet, something inside me told me this might not happen. I started to feel a growing emptiness for the family I had hoped for, and any future pregnancies. What if I could never get pregnant again?

It felt as though my body was telling me to give up, and as Christmas approached feelings of despair and resentment started to build up inside me. For the first time on this journey, I started to feel as though someone was having a laugh at my expense. Surely we had been through enough and experienced ample challenges, so why were we facing yet another hurdle when we had come so close to a solution?

Still I refused to give up, and just waiting it out wasn't an option for me. I knew my 'advanced age' at now thirty-eight was another issue to face, yet with each month passing and no cycle, that biological clock was ticking harder and louder.

After seven months and still no change it was important for my sanity and my relationships to find my own way through this cloud. I searched for reasons why my cycle had not returned. Something was definitely amiss; I could sense it. I knew that time and just waiting would not solve this issue and I was determined to take matters into my own hands. My dream, my destiny was to become a mother, therefore it was up to me to make this a reality.

I scoured the Internet with different searches. Whilst I was now fully aware of the risks of Google in searching for answers, I had no other option, and I was going into this with an open mind. I hit some online forums and asked questions. There had to be something out there that would at least point me in another direction. This lack of knowing was becoming excruciating and I needed to get back some control and find my own answers.

I searched a number of sites, always asking the same question. 'Why has my period not returned seven months following a miscarriage?'

There was one answer that kept popping up in my search, and in my mind it was worth exploring further. Many pointed towards the D&C procedure I had undergone to medically remove the foetus from my body. At the time, the procedure was recommended to me. I had a long and arduous miscarriage after my third loss, with haemorrhaging and two emergency hospital stays. When the fourth loss was found, the hospital advised that a D&C was the best and quickest option to help my body recover from the miscarriage.

I was completely unaware that the procedure came with risks that could impact my fertility. In fact, as I searched, I found a site that quoted a five percent chance of damage to the uterine lining following a D&C, which could ultimately affect future pregnancies and cause infertility. The condition was called 'Asherman's syndrome' and it was considered very rare, and many sites stated that doctors did not even believe it was a serious matter. As I continued my research, I could only find one primary specialist in the UK who advocated management of the condition. From what I could tell, it wasn't something the public system even fully recognised as a condition. Reading this made me feel a little comforted, although scared that I may have this condition; perhaps this could be the reason I wasn't getting my cycle back. Every explanation of the symptoms felt like they were talking about me personally. Again, I had to question, if I did have Asherman's Syndrome, why me? Yet another statistic to add to my repertoire?

I went back to my doctor to seek advice on this condition and ask for a referral to the specialist I'd sourced. My doctor dismissed my research, telling me I was over-reacting and to stay off the Internet. She was probably right, but to be frank, where else could I go at this stage? No one else was giving me any other options to pursue, I suggested to her. We discussed the subject for a while.

"Just wait a little longer dear, your body will eventually rectify itself," she said to me. I could tell she thought I was wasting my time with the referral request.

"Eventually? It's been seven months." I emphasised. "I need to explore this to at least rule it out. I'd like to meet this specialist, please." I pushed, fixing my gaze on her so that she knew I wasn't leaving this office without the referral.

"I really don't recommend it." She almost tutted at me in response, but I refused to give in. This was my body, and it was at no expense of hers to write this referral.

"Look if I'm wrong, at least its another avenue I've explored. I can't sit and wait. I'm not doing this via the public system, I need a private referral." I wasn't leaving her office without that little piece of paper, and I watched as she shook her head and reluctantly turned back to her computer.

She handed me the referral letter, telling me once more that she was sure it would be just a matter of time before I got my period back. I couldn't understand why she seemed so resistant; it was my money and my time that I'd be wasting if I were wrong. I could tell that my doctor thought I was foolish as I left her office with the referral. In fact, as I read her letter I had to laugh at one particular sentence.

'My patient <u>believes</u> she has Asherman's syndrome.'

Perhaps this was leading to another dead end, and my doctor was right, but at least then I could put my mind at ease knowing I had explored the option.

It felt strange when I was eventually proven right. I actually didn't want to be; I had hoped the solution would be much simpler. On the other hand, I had been given a reason why my cycle hadn't returned after seven months.

The specialist found that I had severe scarring throughout my uterus, with blockages and adhesions that were impacting my menstrual cycle and my ability to conceive. Whilst the diagnosis itself didn't solve my problem, at least it assured me that I wasn't going crazy. This wasn't just a waiting game, as I had been told previously. The longer I left this condition, the more permanent it could become.

It was also at this point when I realised the road I was travelling was about to get a whole lot rougher. My new specialist was honest, informative and realistic. Getting pregnant again may not be possible even if I could reverse the damage inside my uterus. I walked away feeling disheartened and robbed by the ineptitude of those surgeons who had performed my original D&C procedure.

The only solution for me now was more surgery, as well as a series of hormone drugs and double the patience. I was also advised that the odds were around fifty percent, at most, of successfully conceiving again, and even then, it was highly likely that I would have problems carrying a baby to full term. Surely it was about time to call it a day?

Yet, something inside me wanted to keep fighting for this. I couldn't give up now. Fifty percent meant there was still a chance. I was ready to take my bet on those odds. If I did walk away, I would never know if the odds would fall in my favour, I had to hope that eventually good fortune would prevail.

Storm Damage

At this point in time, I had been on this road for just on three years, and it started to feel as though I was reaching my emotional crossroad. Both my body and my mind felt tormented by the loss of multiple pregnancies, the frustration of continually trying between those pregnancies, as well as the roller coaster of hormones and emotions that overwhelmed my body as it recovered each time. I felt as though each time I was given a glimpse of hope it was taken away from me, and once again I was facing a dead-end.

As a couple, we were well aware of the other options available to us. One of the options we had discussed at great length was adoption. We even scheduled an appointment with a local social worker who could give us more information. We had a lengthy meeting with this woman in our own home, asked a myriad of questions about the process, our options and even started completing forms.

It was positive to hear that rules around adoption in the United Kingdom were changing, making it now much more accessible and transparent. We went into the discussion under no illusions that this would be a simple process, and we certainly didn't assume we would get a rosy-cheeked newborn from an unwed teenager. Yet, I can honestly say that after three hours with this very straight-talking and sincere social worker, both my husband and I had a lot to think about. The social worker took us through the entire approval and selection process, which would be both intrusive and demanding. We were advised of the potential social, physical and mental backgrounds of many of the children awaiting adoption, and that once a match was found we should expect a prolonged 'settling in' period.

Adoption is a commitment, and it's not for everyone. As a couple, we understood the steadfastness that would be required to provide these children a strong, supportive and stable upbringing. I was open to adoption and exploring it further someday, my husband was less so. We had always agreed that we both had to be one hundred percent or it was nothing at all.

As a couple, we had weighed up the pros and cons, and we didn't feel it was fair to give any false expectations to a child waiting for adoptive parents. What if we did get our chance at having our own baby? We couldn't ignore the fact that there was still a chance. Consequently, we shelved the idea of adoption at this stage, and decided that we had come too far to turn back or stop our original plan. We were open to re-opening a discussion on this course at a later date, but we agreed that our own conception journey was potentially not yet finished.

I had my new specialist lined up, and a potential solution that involved surgery and drugs, but I wasn't ready to start. My body still felt wrecked, and I couldn't shake off my emotions. I felt like I needed some headspace and time to just stop thinking about getting pregnant or being a mother. I couldn't walk into another process feeling the way I did. To be perfectly frank, this was the lowest I had felt on this entire journey. Whilst I realised that time was precious and my biological clock was ticking faster with each month, my own sanity demanded some relief from the process.

I wasn't giving up; I was just pressing the pause button. I had spoken to many women who had been 'trying to conceive' for several years continuously. I could see how the strain had sometimes taken its toll on family, friendships, career, personal life and occasionally rationality. I could see that I was starting to head down a very dark path. I was quick to snap, and becoming cynical and irrational in my reactions to people and situations. I couldn't be that person; it wasn't me, and I had to get back to where I had been before all this heartbreak and discouragement. I wanted to find my true self once again, and then I would be ready for this next chapter.

When, and perhaps even if, I did continue to pursue this path, it was important for me, my husband, and hopefully our rainbow baby, that I would be able to rebalance my mindset. I want to be a good mother, and to do that I need to be a good person. Recognising that I was on a downward spiral of hurt, confusion and, at times, anger about what I had been forced to endure was hard, but ignoring it was not an option.

To be completely honest, once I made this decision I felt liberated. It was as though the relentless pressure I had been placing on myself for so long had suddenly lifted. It was only a few months, but it meant for just a little while I could just stop the counting, sensing, thinking, and lighten the overwhelming burden I was placing on myself to get pregnant.

My plan was to spend some time healing. I needed to reflect and understand my emotions; and in some way, come to terms with my 'lot in life'.

Over the past three years I made it through everything purely through self-preservation. Often I would preoccupy myself with work, social arrangements, exercise and even my writing. I'd find myself putting on a 'happy face' to anyone and everyone. Yet beneath the surface, I knew I was falling apart slowly. There was no doubt in my mind, I did want to start trying again, but getting back to the essence of me was much more important. I had to find my true self again before I could even contemplate commencing the entire conception process again.

With my future as a mother up in the air, it was natural for me to be harbouring many different feelings: anger, resentment, grief, self-pity and hopelessness. However, even though I felt these emotions, I can honestly say I have never felt aggrieved towards others. Naturally, it was difficult at times to hear that others were falling pregnant and starting families, but I could never begrudge them this wonderful milestone in their lives. To wish them anything other than the happiness they deserved would have been incredibly hypocritical of me. After all, one day I truly hoped it would be me sharing that wonderful news with others.

So many times, however, I felt like I was just an observer, an onlooker. Every month I would watch other women who had been blessed fall pregnant quickly and with no problems whatsoever. Of course I envied them. I wanted to be just like them. Snap my fingers and bam I'm pregnant and the entire experience is wonderful and stress free. I wanted to be that woman. I certainly didn't resent their experience, but it did make me question why so many women have to suffer through the pain of infertility, when others have so much ease with the process. Sometimes life does not play a fair game.

Those women, the ones who float through their pregnancy, are so lucky to never have to understand the struggles faced by infertility and pregnancy loss. In talking to many I know they cannot comprehend the anxiety I feel sometimes about falling pregnant again, and facing perhaps yet another loss. Sometimes I hear flippant comments from them, giving me advice for 'next time'. Little do they know I've probably already tried everything that they've suggested. I hold my tongue and nod and smile. I know I was once that naïve and I truly hope that they never have to experience any of it. No one should.

Then, there are the families who have triumphed over their own challenges with infertility, miscarriage, loss or trying to conceive. I've watched in awe as many couples finally reached their destination. My heart fills with them as I watch that immense joy when they finally get to hold the child they've been yearning for. I look to those couples with hope and encouragement; aspiring that one day I will be sharing my own triumph over the beast that is infertility.

Until then, I can only continue to battle through my own struggles, staying focused on my end destination and reminding myself that anything can be possible with a positive mind. Perhaps this sounds a little nonsensical, but then again, this entire experience has never held much logic to me. The 'why me' question remains ever present, and I keep telling myself that perhaps it is Mother Nature's way of telling me that it is not quite our time to be parents. I'm still determined that our time will come, and it is important I remember that, to keep myself on track.

The pain and anger doesn't disappear, but it is now becoming superseded by a determination to overcome this obstacle and reach my own final destination.

It was still raining outside, and I understood that I would need to again face that storm if I wanted to continue this journey. Nevertheless, for now I was happy to stay indoors and allow myself time to recover, dry off and find peace, before once again stepping outside into the weather. Perhaps when that time comes, the storm won't feel so difficult to withstand.

Shaking off the Umbrella

Even though I had embarked on this 'break' from trying to conceive and pregnancy, it was never far from my mind. I had stopped looking for my cycle to return and I felt a little more relaxed as I knew there was nothing I could do until I started treatment. Still, I couldn't shake off the constant reminder that I had to get back on that wagon soon. I tried to focus my energy on other interests, and fortunately it was at this time I signed an agreement to publish my first book. My writing became my outlet, and I was pleased to have something outside of work that could distract me from reality.

At this point, it was now almost nine months since my last period. My final pregnancy's due date, had it been successful, was fast approaching. That finality was ever-present and real. It made me question whether I was being sensible by putting the brakes on trying, and whether I should be kick starting this treatment and surgery. There was nothing stopping me, just my own hesitation and self-preservation.

There was also a question nagging me. Did I really want to put myself through this? The last three years had been one hell of a roller-coaster ride. My body was tired, my emotions were wrought, and now I had this prevailing paranoia that whatever course I did take, something would go wrong. Would my four losses continue to haunt me, creating an unnecessary anxiety to an already stressful time? That was why the time wasn't right to re-start my journey. I knew that I still felt overwhelmed by it all, and I wasn't ready just yet.

Over the following two months I followed through on my personal commitment, focusing all of my energy on me. I knew I wouldn't press pause for too long, but it was long enough to re-ignite the way I wanted to approach this next phase of my fertility journey. I set up a blog, and quite quickly received a following from many others who could share my plight. Each of us were different; we all had stories to tell, but for me it was helpful to make these connections. I found blogging a great outlet to start channelling my feelings and experiences, and the encouragement of other women all over the world inspired me.

In many ways, my writing had become cathartic. I had joined a community of women who shared my frustration, pain and grief; and in doing so I found myself healing. I became inspired by those who had been fighting against their infertility for years, hearing their stories about their setbacks and coping mechanisms, as well as the accounts of those who triumphed against the odds. All this helped me to gain the perspective I needed. I hadn't set a specific timeframe for myself on how long I would wait before moving forward, but by month three, I felt ready to begin again. Something had triggered, and I knew I was in a much better place. Those fears hadn't completely subsided, but I could feel my strength and willpower rebuilding, and I hoped that would be enough to supersede any doubts.

Jointly, my husband also discussed restarting. I could tell he was worried. He had seen me go through four losses and he was concerned that another setback would take its toll on my mental and physical state. Yet, we both agreed that I had to have this procedure, if only to get my menstrual cycle back to normal. We would take each step at a time. The road ahead could still be rocky, but we would face it together.

I was lucky, as soon as I made the appointment with my new specialist the surgical procedure was scheduled within a few weeks; a hysteroscopy which would involve microscopic attention to my poor, battered uterus. The specialist would be able to see first-hand just how much damage had really been done through that

D&C procedure. Hopefully, he would be able to take immediate measures to remove any adhesions, scar tissue or blockages and get me back on the road to trying for a baby. I was very nervous of course, but I was also assured of the expertise of this specialist, and if anyone could help me, this was the person to do so.

Rain Predicted

Many people, who know me well, understand that I'm not one to do things by halves. Once I had booked the surgery I wanted to start off this next chapter with a positive spin. The surgery was booked for the week after Easter, and we were lucky to have a four-day weekend around the holiday. So I convinced my husband that we should take that weekend and go away to the countryside. I wanted to take my mind off the anticipation and nervousness that started rebuilding. I felt that a change of scenery, a little indulgence and some long relaxing walks through the tranquil countryside would help us both. It was perfect.

Then, to top this off, I had also planned a short beach break with two of my girlfriends following the surgery. Again, I knew in advance I would be in recovery, and I'm not a very good patient at the best of times. I needed an excuse to relax, recuperate and do nothing. What could be better than soaking up some sunshine by the beach with a good dose of Vitamin D. To many this may sound a little crazy, but for me it made perfect sense. When I told my surgeon of my plans his expression was that of amusement and shock. Partly because the beach break involved a long flight, albeit I had upgraded my seat, and he did agree that it would at least ensure I was limiting any physical activity and resting.

When the day of my procedure arrived, I was naturally full of butterflies. Although I tried my hardest not to over-think what could or couldn't be following the surgery, it was constantly playing on my mind. For me, I was hedging all my bets on reversing all that damage that had been done following my last miscarriage. I didn't know how I would cope if it didn't work. I had forced myself to think positively up until this point, and I was now in the hands of fate, and this specialist. As I checked into the hospital at six-thirty the morning of my procedure, the fears of what may not be started to arise. My surgeon met me in my small hospital room, empathetically reassuring me that he would do his absolute best to get me 'baby ready'. Fortunately, I was the first on his list that morning, so I didn't have a lot of waiting around.

Within less than an hour of arriving I was prepped for surgery, making it even harder for me to dwell on those fears. I welcomed the cloud of oblivion as the anaesthetist asked me to count down from ten, and trusted that all would be okay from here. It only felt like minutes before I was being woken in the recovery ward. I was disoriented, my mouth was dry and my stomach ached. Loud noises and beeps were all around me as I heard the nurse speaking to me about something. I'm not even sure if I answered her as I tried to regain my senses. I remember being wheeled back to my hospital room through waves of slumber, closing my eyes, but not quite falling asleep.

It's strange how you lose all sorts of dignity in a hospital. As I woke again later, and felt like my consciousness was resuming, I looked around my small room. Thank God there was no one here, as I had ripped off the sheets and I was wearing an unattractive surgical gown, which had unravelled and fallen apart, exposing me to anyone who walked in. My stomach ached and I could see it was slightly bloated. The nurses came in and out of my room regularly to check my temperature and blood pressure. I welcomed a cup of tea and a small bite to eat, suddenly feeling ravenous. As the haze from my anaesthesia slipped away completely, I was becoming more eager to find out how the surgery went; whether it was successful. My husband, who was always by my bedside, urged me to be patient, encouraging me to eat and perhaps get changed into something a little more comfortable. It was several hours post the procedure before my specialist did arrive, and I was dressed, sitting up, and waiting on the side of the hospital bed. He apologised for the delay, but explained he had had a long list of surgeries that day.

As he gave me the news of the outcome, my heart fell. "Fifty-fifty," he told me. He wasn't confident that the procedure was completely successful. He went on to explain that there had been a lot of damage inside my uterus, and that I may need to have a second procedure, or worse case, consider surrogacy. He described my uterus as a spider-web; the scarring and adhesions made it difficult for him to navigate. He did his best to unblock and remove the damage, but only time would tell if it was enough. His words flattened me. *Fifty-fifty!*

He tried to sound encouraging, but his voice told me that he wasn't positive. He explained I would now need to undertake a course of a high dose of oestrogen for the next four weeks, and that he had also inserted a 'coil' which would need to be removed on day twenty-eight exactly. I was advised I had to follow his instructions to the day, and that I should make an appointment with my local doctor to remove the coil. He had scheduled a follow up appointment with me for six weeks, and suggested that if the surgery was a success I should have a menstrual cycle by that stage.

My body needed time to heal. I had to relax and recuperate, and hope. Whilst I knew that nothing was ever guaranteed, I left the hospital feeling disheartened by this news. I was heading towards yet another roadblock. It felt like every time I removed an obstacle, another one popped up further down the path. My husband, ever the supportive companion, encouraged me to look at the fifty percent that was positive, and urged me to try not to over-think it, and just wait and see. Always waiting for something, this was just another test of patience. The reality was that I had no other choice; there was nothing I could do but hope. I was glad now to have this beach holiday in front of me. My friends would certainly take my mind off my current plight, and I would be forced to enjoy the sunshine and banter.

It was only a short break away, but for me it was exactly what the doctor ordered! I came back refreshed and open-minded. My husband was right; I had to focus on the fifty percent chance that it could be a positive result. I was determined to follow the recovery plan laid out to me, and soon enough I would know one way or another. I had to trust that eventually my persistence would pay off with some good news.

Thunder and Lightning

As you wait for time to pass, it seems to go so much slower. Each day is counted out, and you feel like time is literally standing still. Although I did try to put it out of my mind, I found my anticipation growing as I progressed closer to the twenty-eight-day mark.

Over the next twenty-eight days I obediently followed the instructions of my specialist to the letter, taking all of my daily medications and injections. They were arduous and painful but I knew if this turned out to be successful, it would all be worth it. I had meticulously scheduled my doctor's appointment three weeks in advance of day twenty-eight exactly, as instructed by my specialist. I even called the surgery, rather than using the online booking system so that I could advise them of the full reason for my appointment. I wanted to ensure there were no surprises on the day. I was pretty sure they would have received notes from my surgical procedure anyway, but nevertheless, I wanted to be absolutely sure. After hearing my explanation, the receptionist did not object, my appointment was confirmed, and so I was comforted that all was prepared. I wasn't sure exactly what a coil removal entailed, but I assumed it was straightforward from the way my specialist had spoken. I was a little anxious about this process, but my surgeon had assured me that it was a straightforward process and that 'any' doctor could remove it. Now it was just more waiting.

It seemed like an eternity before those three long weeks eventually passed, and I reached the twenty-eighth day. I arrived at my doctor's surgery after work, just in time for my appointment. It felt like I had reached a mini milestone and bizarrely I was excited. In two more weeks I had my follow up appointment with the surgeon, and I would finally know whether his fifty-fifty prediction would swing in my favour. I had convinced myself to remain hopeful!

Entering the consultation room, my doctor was seated at her desk in the middle of the room. She looked up at me, and it was clear to me that she had endured a long day. "Yes, Rachel, how can I help you?" she said in a tired voice.

I had hoped she would read my appointment notes, or at least the hospital summary, but nonetheless I obliged. "I had a hysteroscopy with my specialist four weeks ago, and I'm here as I need the coil removed that was inserted during the procedure." The doctor shook her head at me, looking a little lost. So I continued my explanation, telling her that I had made this appointment three weeks ago on the instruction of my specialist. I told her about my surgery, that I had a coil inserted, and that I'd been advised it should be removed by my doctor on exactly day twenty-eight. I gave her as much detail as I knew about the procedure and what my specialist had told me. She looked at me, not saying anything. I asked her, "Did the hospital send you my surgery notes?"

"No, they did not!" she snapped at me quite abruptly. I was taken aback at her response towards me. I didn't know what to say. It certainly wasn't what I had expected. "How dare you just enter my consulting room expecting me to remove your coil? I'm not sure I'm even comfortable with this, given your history." It felt like an accusation, and I could feel myself getting upset at her indignation. It was as though I had intentionally come in to make her day worse and that my medical history was some kind of disease. I tried to focus on remaining calm; I needed her to remove this coil today.

"I'm sorry. I assumed that the hospital would have sent you the surgical notes. I did give them your details," I justified, trying my best to control the quiver in my voice. "My surgeon told me to have this coil removed at day twenty-eight exactly. That's today. He told me it could be removed by any doctor?"

"Your surgeon cannot assume what I can or cannot do!" Her temper seemed to flare towards me. "Rachel, I have received no information whatsoever from your surgeon." I was so shocked by her outburst. This wasn't what I had planned for at this appointment. It was meant to be a simple process? My specialist had assured me of that. I felt embarrassed and upset by her anger towards me and it felt as though I was the one in the wrong here.

"We could call my surgeon; I have his secretary's number?" I suggested eagerly. I quickly checked my watch and they would still be open, so it was possible.

"I really don't have time for this and I certainly don't feel comfortable with what you're asking me." Her voice was now raised, and I was made to feel like a naughty two-year-old.

Until this point I had kept my emotions controlled, but suddenly everything seemed to flood out of me. The long wait until this very day, anxiety and the anticipation of not knowing if the surgery had been a success, and possibly the immense amount of hormones flowing through me from the medications I had been taking, all seemed to bubble beyond my control. I stood up from the chair I was sitting on as I felt my frustrations boil over.

"I am sorry if this 'inconveniences' you, but this entire experience has been horrendous for me. You know what I've been through!" I pleaded with her. "This surgery was to help me get pregnant. I called and made this appointment three weeks ago, explaining why I was coming in. No one told me you were unable to do this! My surgeon assured me this was straightforward and 'any' doctor could remove my coil. That's why I'm here today. I came to you as my doctor, and you're treating me like I am in the wrong. I have only offered solutions and all you can do is chastise me!" I was almost choking as my tears started flowing, I couldn't help but cry.

The doctor wouldn't even look up at me. She sat staring at her computer, and started typing something. I waited for her to say something, but she didn't. "Tell me what have I done wrong to you today?" I asked her, crying, standing there, and waiting for her to respond. She still didn't respond and kept typing. "I'm sorry. I don't understand why I am at fault here? What have I done wrong?" I repeated, feeling myself get more upset. She didn't even look up. "Hello? Can you please talk to me?" I tried again. I was shaking now with both distress and anger.

"Rachel, I do not feel comfortable removing your coil today," she repeated to me again in a slow, stern voice, talking to me like a child and never looking up from her computer screen. I knew I was emotional and upset, but I couldn't control my crying. It was her reaction to me that had sent me into this state.

"I've done nothing wrong here." I again justified, "I really need this removed today. I have no other option. I'm sorry if I've become upset, but this has just been such an anxious time and all these drugs I'm taking must be making me more emotional." My doctor said nothing. "Please! I need you to remove this today."

"I will not be removing your coil, Rachel," she said sternly.

I broke down into a full flood of tears. I couldn't believe it. I stood there looking at her, but she wouldn't even look at me. I had never been treated this way by anyone, and I still didn't understand what I had done wrong. Realising this woman was not going to budge, I'd had enough.

"I will never be returning to this surgery!" I said to her.

I knew she didn't care. She didn't even look up as I stormed out of that consultation room, still in fits of tears, shaking and humiliated. I ran to my car and sat in the driver's seat trying to control myself. I felt frenetic, as I tried to control my sobs and my breathing. I couldn't even turn on the ignition of my car. Feeling like a fool, I called my husband, who was still at work. When he answered my call, I tried to speak but I could only sob into the phone. He tried to get me to slow down, talk to him. He had no idea what had happened, and I realised I was making him anxious with my frantic call. As I finally breathed, I was able to get a few brief words of explanation. He couldn't do much except console me over the line until I calmed down. I just needed to hear his kind and caring voice.

I sat in that car, parked on the street for over fifteen minutes, until I felt calm enough to drive. However, as soon as I walked through the door, the tears returned in floods again. Every time I replayed the conversation with my doctor I feel anxious and upset. I knew it was probably a build-up to this moment, but I also felt that she had treated me with unfair contempt, and I still didn't understand why.

On top of that, I still needed to get this coil removed and I had to regain some of the control I'd lost to find someone who could help. I was comforted when my husband arrived home from work early, and finally I could explain to him in detail what had happened. I cried throughout my story, and he consoled me. Of course he would always take my side, but he was genuinely angry at the way I had been treated in that doctor's office. I couldn't help but replay the events over, trying to think if I could have managed it any differently. I regretted getting so emotional in front of her, but it wasn't as though she hadn't provoked my outburst.

With the help of my husband, we found an out-of-hours doctor service that was nearby, and I was able to get an appointment for the next morning. Fearful of repeating the events, I explained in detail what the appointment was for, and asked the receptionist if she wouldn't mind checking personally with the doctor if there would be any issues with removing my coil. The receptionist was understanding, and promised to call me back once she had confirmed the appointment details with the doctor. Within thirty minutes, she did call back, stating that there would be no issue with removing my coil, and that the doctor would be pleased to see me in the morning. I relaxed a little; at least that was one thing off my mind.

I barely slept that night, waking up as my mind continued to go over that awful experience with my doctor. I would find myself tearing up as I could hear her voice over and over in my head. When I did sleep, I found myself having dreams about it, nightmares in fact. It was an anxiety I had never really felt before and I couldn't shake it. I knew my emotions were heightened anyway, but I also started to wonder why I always seemed to face such adversity through this journey. In the early hours of the morning I sent a note to the receptionist of my specialist, knowing, of course, she wouldn't receive it until she arrived in the office. I told her of the situation with my doctor, that the surgical notes had not been sent by the hospital, and also of her refusal to remove my coil. I was desperate to know if I had in fact done anything wrong here.

The next morning I was tired and drained. My appointment was at eight o'clock with this new doctor, and not wanting to be late I set off extra early. I was actually shocked at how smooth the appointment was. The doctor I met with was a kind lady, who quickly removed my coil, explaining that it was quite a straightforward procedure. I told her briefly about my local doctor's reaction the day before, and she seemed more baffled than I was.

"I'm not sure why she couldn't remove your coil. It's a fairly straightforward procedure," she told me.

I shrugged. I couldn't speak, as I knew if I did I'd just start crying again.

By the time I got home, I had an email from my specialist in my inbox. He apologised for the surgical notes not reaching my doctor, and he stated his confusion at the issue with my doctor. He advised that he'd never heard of a doctor refusing to remove a coil before. It reassured me a little to know that I wasn't in the wrong, and I was even more relieved to know that the coil was now removed.

The stress and anxiety of the twenty-four hours that had passed weighed on me heavily, and unable to even contemplate returning to work that day I decided to try to finally get some sleep. I was still highly distressed by the experience, but I forced myself to put it to the back of my mind, focusing on getting through the next two weeks. All would hopefully reveal itself then, and hopefully now the worst part was over!

Once I had reflected on the events that had played out, I decided I would register with a new doctor. I felt disappointed by my local doctor's response, and regardless of whether she was having a bad day, or just felt aggrieved that she didn't have my surgery notes, I was still upset. I didn't deserve her retaliation against me, and I expected more support and empathy from a medical professional. They could transfer my notes and my history, and I was hoping that from here on, I would have more fortune with my plans to become a mother. It was time for a fresh, new start!

A Break in the Rain

Unfortunately, when I returned to the specialist the news wasn't positive. The surgery didn't work, and whilst a scan revealed some improvement, I would need a further surgical procedure. My period hadn't returned, and it should have by now, and there were no signs that the blockages in my uterus had cleared. My specialist explained to me that he had expected this; that during the procedure he could barely get access to my uterus through the adhesions and scarring.

It was recommended that I undergo the same procedure again, and whilst my heart fell, I was told that in my case it could take multiple procedures to get back to normal. Whatever normal is now? I agreed, and scheduled myself in as quickly as possible. There was no more waiting, and I could only move forward. The specialist was slightly more positive this time after my procedure, but did warn me that given the extent of the damage in my uterus, there was a chance the adhesions and scarring could re-form. For the following month I was back on the medications and injections. I felt bloated from the hormones I was taking, and my stomach was heavily bruised from the blood thinning injections I had to take daily. It was another twenty-eight-day wait, but this time I returned to my specialist for the removal of that coil. I wasn't prepared to risk another incident, even though I had a new local doctor set up.

Six weeks after my second surgery, I hoped and prayed that my cycle would return, indicating that the surgery had worked. My specialist had assured me, 'any time now'.

Well, lo and behold, a few days later, it was there. I was ecstatic. My first period in twelve months! Truth be told, it was incredibly light, and lasted a few hours at most, but it was there, and I had convinced myself it was a positive sign of things to come. I'm not sure I know of anyone who was so excited to see their period arrive. Nonetheless, this was a significant milestone for me, and I felt one step closer to where I needed to be on this journey. I suddenly felt as though a heavy weight had been lifted off my chest.

When I returned to the specialist once again, the scan showed an improvement in my uterine lining. But I could tell immediately by his tone that the outcome wasn't as positive as I had hoped. As he examined me, I was told that he had expected to see more improvement and there were still signs of scarring and adhesions. In his small consultancy room, he had a large screen monitor which I could watch as he conducted my scan. It was all black and white squiggles to me, but as he talked me through them, it was obvious the results weren't brilliant. He did sight a small follicle, and suggested that we might try to conceive naturally over the coming week. I could tell from his voice that the chances of a pregnancy were slim, but still I agreed to follow his instruction. We set a follow up an appointment for another six weeks, and decided we would discuss a third surgery at that point in time if there was no pregnancy.

I wanted to remain positive, set on believing that the odds could fall in our favour. My husband and I resolved to give it our best shot. I may sound a little naïve at times, but positivity was the only way forward on this journey. Going into this half-hearted wasn't going to get us anywhere, and it had now been over twelve months since my last pregnancy, I refused to believe that I wouldn't fall pregnant ever again.

It was strange getting back into the mindset of *trying to conceive* again. We hadn't really thought about it much for almost six months; we couldn't! Planning and timing had gone out the window due to my body's refusal to menstruate. We had enjoyed the spontaneity for a period of time, as well as the breather from counting days, checking for ovulation patterns and symptoms. It felt strange being back on that wagon.

To top off the pressure, this was not just any monthly cycle; this was the one after the surgery, which would hopefully return my body to normal. I felt immensely apprehensive as I wanted and hoped that either way my body would show me it was also fighting for this cause.

Alas, this particular battle was not the one I would win. I tested for a possible pregnancy every day leading up to my supposed end of cycle date. The test remained stark blank with just the one control line. I had led myself to believe I was experiencing possible early pregnancy signs, but as each day progressed my hopes were getting dimmer. Our little bathroom bin was quickly filled with used, negative tests; and even worse, my period hadn't even arrived. The signs weren't looking good either way.

I waited another two weeks, and knowing I definitely wasn't pregnant, I became even more fearful that my cycle hadn't rectified itself. I felt like I was going back to square one. I finally yielded. Letting go of the unwavering optimism I had been holding onto I scheduled a follow up appointment with my specialist. One step forward, two steps back. I should be used to this now, but each setback still seemed to take the wind out of me.

        This journey was certainly testing my will power and determination. Still, I am a fighter, and this battle was not yet over!

Wet Weather Blues

Infertility is a Bitch. It's a big and nasty BITCH, all in capital letters. It had to be said before I keep going, and frankly, I'm just saying what we all think. If you're going through any type of infertility challenges, I'm sure you'd support my viewpoint. It just sucks. It's indiscriminate, it's unfair and sometimes it's unforgiving.

Why me? Why anyone? Over the years I've researched the hell out of infertility, miscarriages and all and sundry about problems trying to conceive or carry a baby. From what I can tell, there doesn't seem to be a straightforward answer to any of it. It's not just age, it's not always lifestyle choices and there's no particular pattern towards its victims – it sometimes feels all a bit random.

I am constantly being told that it is just about my age, that this is the primary reason for my issues, that I started trying for a baby too late. It's not just my doctors who are telling me this too. It's all around me, in everything I read. But really, is it? I know many people in their early twenties, as well as those whose lifestyles couldn't be any healthier with exercise and a well-balanced diet, who have also struggled to conceive and carry a baby. I also know people who live a polar opposite lifestyle, who have had no issues whatsoever conceiving and enjoying a straightforward pregnancy. For me, there doesn't seem to be one factor that causes it all. That's the toughest thing to get my head around. When I ask myself what could I have done differently, I really don't know if there is an exact answer.

     The biggest problem for me is this holding pattern that I've been standing in for now four years. Every decision I have made has been based around a question mark of whether I will or won't be pregnant. I'm on stop-start mode constantly. Today I can exercise, tomorrow I can't. Today I can book that holiday, organise that event or go out and enjoy myself, but tomorrow I need to rest, recuperate or just wait for a result that may not be. My body feels all over the place; I'm no longer the person I was, and I feel all out of sorts. When I look at myself in the mirror, I know I'm not the person I used to be, and physically I feel bloated and gross; I'm just not myself. Despite trying my best to keep healthy and stay fit, I just don't feel it anymore. Worse still, I've actually stopped caring.

It was only recently when I was getting ready to go to a friend's party when I really took a good look at myself. I threw on a pair of jeans (which were bordering on too tight) and a loose top to cover my bloated belly (which felt so uncomfortable from all those meds). As I was pulling my hair up into a messy ponytail, I looked in the mirror and I was shocked at the person I'd suddenly become. My face was blotchy and pale, my hair limp and lifeless (most of it had been falling out from my hormone rollercoaster) and I just looked tired and weary. I'd forgotten myself! I had become that woman I never wanted to be. I had lost confidence in myself and I didn't feel good about who I was anymore – physically and emotionally.

So how do I get back to me? How do I reverse this trend, and start to feel good about myself again? It was then I realised that a real change was needed and I had to take back control. In reality, I was still going to ride this rollercoaster, and keep trying for our rainbow baby, but at the same time I needed to stop and take a hard look at myself, my habits and my attitude towards myself and my body. I needed to rebuild my own confidence and reignite myself back to where I was a few years back. If my mind wasn't in the right place, I'd never be ready to have a baby. Suddenly, it wasn't only my mindset on the line; it was my future as a mother.

Only then, after a good hard look at my life, could I see that at this point in time I was not in the best state to become a mother. Every waking thought had become about getting pregnant, but what I had forgotten was the true purpose of this quest. Above everything, I had to be a fit, happy and healthy mum. I had to be everything for that child if we were blessed with our rainbow baby, and right now, I wasn't even happy with myself.

As I looked in my mirror, getting ready to go out, I made a pact with myself. I would turn this all around and it had to start now. I would find ways around the restrictions placed on me, and I would stop making excuses for myself. I refused to stand in front of that mirror tomorrow feeling sorry for myself. Only I could control my destiny, and I was going to have my rainbow baby one day. When that day finally arrived, I wanted to be the best mum I could be, both physically and emotionally.

Knee Deep in Rain Puddles

Reaching that twelve-month mark since our last pregnancy was difficult, and finding out that we were still no further along was even harder.

I'm sure anyone else who has suffered pregnancy loss is the same; there are certain milestones and dates that are never far from our thoughts. Sadly, I remember them all. Sometimes I would keep my thoughts to myself as due dates approached, reflecting on what might have been. Whilst I've tried to focus on looking forward, sometimes I need to look back too, as I think about those four little angels I was never able to hold. My pregnancies had never progressed far enough to even find out their gender. Those little foetuses were barely formed, millimetres in size, yet still they were important to me. Perhaps some find my sentimentality a little bizarre, but to me they held significance. They were the hope of a family I had dreamed of having.

At this point, I felt my optimism wavering, as I met again with my specialist who suggested a third procedure. I had to ask myself how much more I could endure. Each surgery involved a recovery period, and surely my body could only withstand so much? I agreed to the surgery, but this time around I didn't feel as positive. In my mind, this would have to be my last chance to fix the damage that had been done; and then what?

It wasn't fair to my husband, either. We were heading into our fourth year of trying to conceive, losses, heartbreak, medical examinations, and the rollercoaster of emotions that come with it. I could only imagine how he must have felt as he watched me go through it all. Even if the surgery did work, we were never guaranteed that a pregnancy would even be successful. Our lives had been consumed by this journey now for too long, there had to be a point where we stopped and looked for another destination. With the date for this procedure approaching, I had also started contemplating my options, preparing myself mentally should I need to reassess our future.

Perhaps this sounds quite melancholy. Nonetheless, I had to approach this next step with common sense. As I prepared myself for this third (and last) surgery, I also needed to be realistic. My body may not cooperate, and it may never be repaired to the extent that I can conceive and carry a child to full term. It was only sensible to start considering how I would cope if my dreams of having a child *naturally* may never come to fruition.

It was also important that my husband and I put our relationship first, above everything else. We were not prepared to go through a myriad of additional and extensive procedures, different medications and then forcing pressure on ourselves to achieve something that Mother Nature was clearly not willing to budge on. We had to set our limits, and this procedure would have to be the stopping point. Worst case scenario, if it didn't work, we were now prepared to walk away from this particular path. We had to; for our sanity, our health, our emotional well-being, and most of all for our future together as husband and wife!

I know how fortunate I am to have such a supportive and caring husband. I wasn't prepared to risk our relationship. If we were walking away from our options to become parents through pregnancy, I wanted to be sure that we still held the same love and affection for each other regardless of the outcome. We had been strong so far, but I wasn't prepared to test how far we could push our limits.

Many times I had contemplated how much was enough? How far could I travel along this road, and when would I know that I couldn't keep going? Deep down, I knew that I was approaching this surgery with the right mindset. Strangely, in making this decision, I felt released, not sad. To me, I had given myself a clear direction. I would go one way and keep walking should this surgery result in success – and I still hoped it would. Yet, if it wasn't a success, I had accepted that exploring a new and different path would also be another adventure I would wholeheartedly and positively discover. I was preparing myself for the worst; I needed to be realistic. I was going in with my eyes wide open and limiting my expectations.

As a couple, we hadn't yet discussed specific alternative options should this surgery fail. There would be plenty to think about, but we decided to wait until this third and last surgery before deciding where to next. For the first time in a while, I felt as though I had regained some control over my destiny. I was standing at a crossroad, and I had two different directions to turn. I wasn't going to let Mother Nature beat me down. It felt both empowered and grateful for this newfound strength as I prepared myself to face the next month with an open mind.

At this time, summer had finally arrived in Britain, and throughout all of this, work had been particularly hectic. I needed a break, some time out from the day to day happenings in life, and so we decided to take a well earned holiday on the South West coast of England before my next surgery. We were still steadfast on our plans, but this was a nice way of spending time with my husband and my dog on the coastline, getting me relaxed and ready for this next important phase of our journey.

If this was successful, I could be back on track and trying for a baby in the next few months. Our life would, of course, change substantially if that were the case. Decisions about my career and life choices would be different, and even the impact of a newborn in our household would mean significant changes. All of those thoughts excited and daunted me. I didn't dare think too much about it, for fear of creating a false expectation.

Over the years I had always known this would be the case. We were prepared for these changes, knowing that impromptu nights out, holidaying and other lifestyle decisions would all change with parenthood. However, now we had to consider the other option. What if our lifestyle didn't change? If we were never to become parents, we would remain on this path. There would be no need for planning for school funding, package family holidays or even school drop offs. All of those things that

I had hoped would be the parenting challenges we'd face, could all disappear if the surgery wasn't successful.

I had to force myself to think that way, to dare to contemplate how we would face that life. I had been spending almost four years trying and planning for a child, as though one day it would be a sure thing. If that road reached a dead-end, I wanted to ensure that my life wasn't lived in regret of what couldn't be. We would be adventurous, career-focused and we would find other ways to fulfil our lives. Regardless of the outcome, I was prepared to face the future head on, to let life take me whichever way the wind blows. It was that freedom in thinking that helped put me in a much better and more positive place to approach this next chapter.

If we were faced with spending the rest of our life without children, I was determined to become the couple we were before this crazy baby-making endeavour. I felt excited and scared about the possibility, but for the first time, I had truly prepared myself for what could inevitably be our future. We would again be the couple who were spontaneous and carefree.

In our little cottage by the sea, we enjoyed a relaxing week away full of long beach walks, lunches sitting on terrace bars, glasses of wine and delicious

Cornish cream teas. With no real agenda or plans, this was exactly what the doctor ordered.

We were lucky to have blue skies and sunshine all week long. Bringing our young dog with us made for a different holiday, as we had to plan out our journey and our days, ensuring that all activities were *doggie friendly.* It helped me gain perspective, knowing that whilst we didn't have children in our family today; we were still a family unit. Our little furry boy has genuinely been a wonderful addition to our household. We decided to adopt him after my third miscarriage, and neither of us has ever regretted that decision. Not even when he barks in the middle of the night or chews a piece of furniture.

At the time, the frustration of three losses and no solutions had us talking about what we could do to appease our pain. I always wanted a dog, and my husband (a non-dog person) finally agreed. Meanwhile, we had still intended on having a baby and continuing to try, and we had carefully thought through the timing of adopting a puppy, knowing that even if our circumstances did change, he would be at least twelve months old before a baby was born.

Alas, it is still the three of us, but our home feels richer with the addition of our little dog, and he literally has both of us wrapped around his little paws. Whatever our future may hold, this dog has also taught us that love can come in a number of different forms, and should our future hold no 'human' children, we can, of course, find an unconventional love with this little man, and perhaps another sibling or two.

The positive side of all of this is that we know we have options. Both my husband and I agreed that we had finally reached certain contentment with what could be an alternative future. If our quest to get pregnant and start a family never reached its final destination, our hearts would survive the pain, and love and happiness still prevail.

We enjoyed our week away in the sunshine, and I felt confident I had the energy to face our next chapter head on.

'Do not go where the path may lead, go instead where this is no path and leave a trail' – Ralph Waldo Emerson.

Storm Chaser

There was no more hiding from it, and certainly no more procrastination; there was only one way forward. Standing still was only keeping me in limbo – it was time to finally get the real answers.

I returned from holiday with only a week until my surgery. I had also decided to fly home to Brisbane not long after the procedure, to spend time with family and recuperate with more sunshine. Some may think I'm slightly mad for booking the long haul flight back home. For me, it would help me through that long wait after the procedure and occupy my time with the distraction of family and old friends.

Sadly, I was well versed with hospital procedures, and I knew my body well, what it could and couldn't do, and the flight didn't worry me. In fact, it was a great excuse to sit still for a dozen or so hours at a time and just watch in-flight movies. It also gave me something to look forward to after the procedure.

When I do think about the number of hospital visits, specialist and doctor's appointments, scans, tests and other medical procedures I've undergone in the past few years, it dumbfounds me. If they awarded mileage points, I'd be on a first class trip around the world! As my husband and I checked into that hospital on the day of my surgery, I felt a sense of déjà vu. Blood pressure, check; weight, check; had any food or drink in the last twelve hours; none, and finally getting dressed into that unattractive and oversized hospital gown; yes, the one with the large gaping backside! It was the same old routine as before. It was a routine I was well used to, but still it didn't make me any less nervous. The nurses and doctors were all very understanding; but then, I guess taking the private specialist and hospital route makes a big difference!

The surgery felt quite straightforward. I was walked into the small operating theatre and then woke up in a daze to be quickly wheeled back to my private little hospital room. My body wanted to keep drifting into an anaesthetically induced sleep but I was also desperate to also find out the news.... *Did it work this time?*

My husband and I waited in my small hospital bedroom, watching whatever daytime television show was being aired, as we eagerly waited the arrival of my specialist with his post-surgery summary. I was wide-awake, despite being under anaesthetic only an hour or so before. It was the adrenalin and anxiety of waiting to find out that had me on tenterhooks. Neither of us really spoke. We were both nervous, and just wanted to know either way.

It was late afternoon before we heard the small knock on the hospital room door, and both of us watched in anticipation as my specialist entered the room. He was still dressed all in blue. It had been a long day; I could see it in his eyes. I sat up straight and my husband grasped my hand with a little squeeze.

"It went beautifully!" My surgeon's words were immediate and amazingly gratifying! He smiled warmly and nodded encouragingly at both of us. I breathed a sigh of relief, feeling my heart pound in excitement. I could tell from his expression that he was being earnest and was immensely satisfied with how the procedure had gone. 'Beautifully' was much better than fifty-fifty and I couldn't have been happier hearing those words at that moment in time!

"Thank you!" I said with all of my heart.

He came to stand beside me and pulled out some scans. I wasn't really sure what I was looking at, but he quickly explained to me the before and after, and I understood that he felt very positive about the way forward. He said there was no reason why my menstrual cycle should not return now. He assured me that this surgery had been much more successful than the last two and he was very confident.

If he was confident, then so was I. I understood there were no guarantees, and even if my menstrual cycle did return, the next challenge would be getting pregnant and staying pregnant. However, at last we were one step closer to our end goal, and this was the news I needed to hear, to keep my hope alive.

Once again I was thrown into another waiting game, with a further four weeks of medicines, injections and hormones to ensure this surgery would sustain the successful results we had hoped for. We agreed to schedule a follow up appointment for the end of August, and hopefully confirm some positive results.

Two days later, I happily relaxed into the long-haul flight to Australia. I felt relaxed and positive, knowing that everything possible was heading in the right direction to get me out of this storm!

I have been living in the United Kingdom now for eight years, and going home to Australia is always something I look forward to. Unfortunately, given the distance and cost, it is not easy getting back and forth as often as I'd like. However, when I do go home, I make the most of reconnecting with friends, family and of course, enjoying the sunshine! This trip, in particular, was a welcome diversion from reality during another four-week wait!

It was difficult, of course, to keep my mind off my personal situation. That glimmer of hope, given to us by my specialist, kept playing on my mind. Whilst I felt more confident with this surgery, I also feared the disappointment of another setback if he was proven wrong. Arriving in Australia my agenda was completely full, and I was lucky as my parents live a street away from the beach, so when I wasn't relaxing with friends I was able to recuperate with a walk by the seaside, or even some writing.

I was committed that I wouldn't over-do it. Whilst I love spending time with friends I've not seen for months, sometimes years, I was also conscious that my body needed to heal, and I wasn't prepared to risk the success of this surgery. I was happy to have quieter nights in with my parents, and whilst it was the end of their winter, the days were still warm, and so it was the perfect environment enjoy the outdoors, or spend the time in front of my laptop creating new blog posts, or even planning my next book.

Writing had become an enjoyable hobby for me, and I found solace in getting lost in my own thoughts and imagination; it helped me take my mind off the reality. I had taken to starting up my journal once again, and publishing pieces on my blog. Writing in some respects had given me the opportunity to take the part of my heart that had closed off with grief and pain, and re-open it to new and different possibilities. My fertility journey was something I wanted to share publicly, to connect with other women, and hopefully let them know they weren't alone in their frustration and pain. Never had I dreamed that my first memoir would ever be published, and the response I received from its publicity was overwhelming. I always hoped I could write a follow up story, something that had a more positive ending. Well, here's hoping!

At this moment, I can't predict the twists and turns of my own story, as I would a fiction novel. I would love to believe I can guide it, but Mother Nature sometimes has a mind of her own. Therefore, I have to let my own chapters unfold with each new day. But will I get my happy ending? Truly that is up to me, whatever the outcome of my surgery. I can't steer my own destiny, but I can choose to embrace it or reject it.

At this moment I therefore choose to embrace whatever life offers me.

Which Way the Wind Blows

Thankfully the weeks didn't feel as long this time. With my trip home to Australia, work, travel and other social events, I found myself reaching the twenty-eighth day once again quicker than I had expected.

Arriving at my follow up appointment, I was glad to be finally finishing the medications and injections, hoping that this would be the last I would see of them. My body felt bloated and bruised, and I knew my emotions were a little sensitive from the hormones I had been taking. My only hope was that the specialist would finally give me the green light to move to the next phase: trying to conceive. Whilst my last interaction with him following the surgery was positive, I still had fears and doubts circling around in my head. Nothing so far had been easy for me, and I could only pray that lady luck was sitting on my side for a change.

My specialist didn't hold me in suspense. As he conducted the scan he immediately told me that everything looked much better than it had previously, and that the results were promising for me. He advised I should stop all medications and I should get a full period within the next two weeks. Based on that, he gave me the go-ahead to start trying again. Finally, we had the news we'd been waiting for!

Then came the warning! I was just now thirty-nine, and due to my advanced maternal age, four miscarriages, and the problems I'd experienced with my uterus, he explained that a natural pregnancy may not be the best possible course. His advice was that I should consider IVF over a natural pregnancy; giving us a greater guarantee of a successful pregnancy. Essentially, he was telling me we could fall pregnant naturally, but did I want to risk another miscarriage – given my age? I felt myself suddenly hitting another fork in the road. Do I let Mother Nature decide the fate of our unborn child, or do I use the genius of science to give us the best chance possible?

IVF was always something I had contemplated might be a future option for us. I knew my age may lead me down this path, but had hoped that since I had fallen pregnant naturally and quite easily in the past it would not be an option we needed to face. We did explore IVF as an option over a year ago; we even made an appointment with a consultant. However, before we could take any further steps, we had fallen pregnant. Unfortunately, like the three others before, that pregnancy didn't last. Now, here we are again today, discussing it as an option.

The thing is, I wasn't sure then, and I'm still not sure now. There is, of course, the cost, but it's much more than that. For me, it's also the physical and emotional strain of the process that scares me. Of course, I'd do anything to have my baby, but how much am I willing to sacrifice based on a 'chance'. As my specialist described his recommendations, those fears re-emerged. We wouldn't have the standard IVF, as getting pregnant wasn't expected to be the issue. We'd have to undergo a certain process of genetic analysis and screening. I would have my body stimulated to produce enough eggs for retrieval; then there would be a hospital procedure to retrieve my eggs, as well as then the process of implantation. On top of this, there would be follow up medications and investigations. Still, there was no guarantee that it would all work.

The cost of all this was significant; in fact, it was double the standard IVF cost. Don't get me wrong, it's not just about money, but with no guarantees it would put a strain on both of us if it failed. Perhaps I was looking at the entire process pessimistically, but I had to be realistic. I've seen relationships stall through this process. I've seen the heartbreak of failed treatments and the costs accumulating with multiple attempts for success. That is a huge concern for me. Round one may not work, so how many times do you keep going back? On top of that, I have seen what it does to the emotional and physical state of those undergoing treatments. At the same time, I know there is a chance it would work, and in fact if it did, the chances of the pregnancy being successful are much higher.

I am confident all of this would be worth it in the long run to hold that lovely baby in our arms. But nothing is guaranteed.

Only a week ago, we had agreed that if our fate meant that we could not have children, and this surgery had not worked, we would accept that. Now it felt as though we were taking this quest for parenthood to another level, a level that may even put more pressure on us to achieve a pregnancy. It felt like two different extremes, and through all this, there was still a chance that I could fall pregnant naturally.

My specialist kept emphasising that my 'advanced' age would be our biggest hurdle now. I'm thirty-nine for Heaven's sake, and I'm still fit, active and healthy. I know the clock is ticking, but I also know others who have had successful pregnancies in their forties. Surely, my time isn't quite gone yet? Perhaps I'm over-exaggerating the quandary we are in, or even over-thinking my options, but I really feel that I still have time on my hands here. Maybe I'm just deluding myself.

For me, a natural pregnancy was still my preferred option. The three of us, me, my husband and my specialist, discussed our options in details. I stood firm. We would see first if my cycle did return, and if so, we'd try naturally for a baby. It was the end of August, and we agreed to give ourselves until December to try it the natural way. If that didn't work, or worse case, we do get pregnant but miscarry again, we would seriously reconsider IVF as a next and final step.

I could tell my specialist didn't fully agree with our decision, but he accepted our choice. We set a follow up appointment with him for early January, and he earnestly wished us luck, hoping that he would see us pregnant at our next meeting.

As we left, both my husband and I knew that there is now a question mark hanging over our heads, as we steadfastly pursue this natural route. Perhaps we are taking a bigger chance on our future baby plans by postponing IVF, but we are not closing that door completely. If we don't try this first, we will always wonder if a natural pregnancy could be possible. Selfishly, we preferred to avoid spending the money, going through pain, emotions, physical stress and medical procedures. My body still felt overwhelmed by three surgeries this year alone. This was the right way forward, and we would get to Christmas and start the New Year either pregnant, or deciding on how to get pregnant via IVF. We had a plan!

The Might of Mother Nature

Within just one week of meeting with my specialist I finally got my period, and it was a real period! I knew this time it was different, as it felt right; it felt normal.

Throughout this entire experience and the last four years, I've realised just how powerful Mother Nature can be. She is a force never to be underestimated. I've been held to ransom by her power, and I accept that. Finally having my period return was a small milestone on a very long journey. It had been well over twelve months since my first full cycle, and I could only pray that everything was back on track.

The weight of the stress, pain, medical procedures and everything else I had been through this year suddenly felt like it was lifted. I had fought so hard, and so long, and finally I felt like I could dare to hope again. Perhaps this could happen?

It was hard to stop myself thinking too far ahead, as suddenly my imagination started to dream of being pregnant again. That was something I had started to shelve away months ago. However, perhaps this could be more than just a dream; perhaps it would be our reality. I was well aware that the road ahead wouldn't be easy, but I had to celebrate these small wins; they kept me going amidst all the setbacks.

So, what to do from here? Well it was still a waiting game and you would think I should be well used to waiting by now. My specialist had advised us *not to try* on this first cycle. He was adamant that we should give my body time and allow it to complete one full menstrual cycle, and take all precautions to avoid a pregnancy. I have to admit, that was hard to contemplate. After all this time, I was ready to go. I wanted to kick things off. But, I knew I had to be careful. So far, I hadn't had a lot of luck in this game, and I didn't want to risk another setback, and ruin my chances. It was just one more month. I'd waited this long, another twenty-eight days wasn't going be the end of the world.

One day I hoped to reflect on this entire journey, to look back and know that it had been worth all the pain and heartbreak. I had been given this chance to try again, and I was determined now to get pregnant by year-end.

Whilst that was a milestone alone, I knew that even if we got pregnant, there would be more hurdles to jump over. But I wanted the chance to jump them, and I hoped Mother Nature would finally work with me, not against me.

I was now doing everything I could to prepare my body for a possible pregnancy. I wasn't going to give Mother Nature any excuse to take this away from me. My diet, my lifestyle, my mindset, were all aligned; I was ready and willing. The only thing I couldn't control was my age, and time was my biggest enemy in this process. Next year, I would be turning forty, and I was well aware I could not waste any opportunity to try to 'get pregnant', as soon as I was able.

Past experience had shown that we could fall pregnant easily. However, we were over twelve months on since our last successful conception, and three surgeries later. Things may prove more difficult. Whilst I still hoped we could get pregnant without assistance, I was not going to wait several months before seeking help. Every step towards my fortieth birthday was reducing the guarantee that we would have a successful pregnancy to full term. I felt like a ticking time bomb.

During those twenty-eight days I had all the signs of a healthy cycle. I even tested for ovulation, and the tests were positive, I was on track. Naturally, we used protection, and followed the orders of my specialist to avoid pregnancy until I'd completed the full twenty-eight days. However, it reinforced my hope and positivity, and on day twenty-seven of my cycle I had another full period. Things were certainly looking good.

By the very end of September, we were ready to go! The official green light on 'trying to conceive' was glowing brightly, and I felt excited and petrified at the same time. I didn't want to bank all of my expectations on this first month of trying, but it was to stop over-thinking everything once again. I was well versed in how to manage my cycle through to conception, but as we started planning out the days I started to ask myself many questions. Was it enough? Should I do something different this time? How will I feel if I do actually fall pregnant? More so, how would I cope in those first few weeks of pregnancy if we do find success? And so it begins . . .

To appease the anxiety, we booked a weekend away in the Cotswold's, a small boutique hotel that would give us the perfect excuse to enjoy each other's company and timed perfectly for my cycle. We needed to relax and take away the pressure of trying to control and plan this next phase. The weather was perfect for walking and exploring, and some quality time together as a couple.

With ovulation there is a very small window, sometimes less than forty-eight hours, and then it is up to Mother Nature to do the rest. As we were back on this path, the many memories of trying in the past came flooding back, and that thought that comes to mind: *Have we done enough to get pregnant this month?*

We hadn't told many people we were starting to try again, but those we did were supportive. It is funny, as suddenly we started to receive all kinds of advice and hints on how to get pregnant; like we had never tried before. One comment in particular always made me smirk: 'Relax, don't think about it and it'll just happen.' Honestly? That statement is completely crazy; how do you stop thinking about it? Especially after everything we've been through. I'm not sure I have the ability to just switch off that part of my brain as much as I would love to.

Then we start the *two-week-wait*: the time between ovulation and menstruation. I'm quickly feeling like the past is coming back to haunt me. Every ounce of my psyche is trying desperately to keep my mind on anything else other than, how many days are left before I can do a pregnancy test? Even worse, I'm not even one hundred percent sure that I got our timing right in the first place. My body has been a little strange, and I can't even guarantee that I did ovulate on time.

As I try to avoid over-analysing supposed symptoms during this agonising two weeks, I find myself becoming frustrated with myself once again. I'm banking too much on this! Relax? I wish!

So why can't I relax? It's that one thought that keeps circling around in my head. I could be pregnant. After all this time, what if this did actually work? It is both strange and exciting, as it just feels so surreal. Just over a month ago, my husband and I had been contemplating our life without children; and now we were getting a chance to change that. To be given that chance again, to just hope that this time it might actually be the real thing. Butterflies flutter in my stomach at the mere thought.

It does make me wonder how so many other women cope with the process of trying to conceive. It is such an emotional journey, and there really is no way of protecting ourselves from the unpredictability of it all. We all hope that it will be an easy road, but for many it is months of trying and waiting, setbacks and losses. I truly hope that soon I will be writing about the joys of pregnancy, and I wonder to myself what it might be like as my belly becomes rounder and I start to feel that little baby move inside me.

I even dare to dream that one day I will be holding my own baby in my arms, watching my husband's reaction as he meets our child for the very first time. It is only my hope that holds this dream alive and keeps me going even through the toughest and darkest moments. Without hope, I would never have had the courage to keep pushing forward; I know that failure is a possibility, but I'm still determined to beat the odds.

At the end of it all, and when this road ends, I am hopeful that **hope will win!**

A Strike of Lightning

Sometimes life just throws you a curve ball from left field. When I least expected it, I'd turn around, and **WHAM,** life has smacked me right between the eyes; completely throwing me off centre. Perhaps I was too engrossed in my own situation, but it was news from my family in Australia that caught me completely by surprise.

My father had cancer! Yes, the big 'C'. It's that word and the diagnosis itself; it sends chills down your spine, as you realise that everything from here on would change. I had only been there just over two months ago, and whilst I could see he had difficulty breathing, I never expected this.

I'm not sure you can ever prepare yourself for this news. Of course, like many of us, I've seen and dealt with cancer before, through family, friends and loved ones. Every time it has caught me off guard. There is nothing nice to say here, cancer is an awful, cruel disease, and the prognosis for my father wasn't good. The doctor said that it was stage four lung cancer, that it was terminal, and I'm utterly powerless to help him. Hearing this, made me think about life and its fragility; that every moment should be cherished, and shouldn't be wasted. But still, this is my dad! Stage four cancer wasn't good on any level. He would need treatment, but there was no cure, it was only prolonging the inevitable. Something I just couldn't fathom. This was my daddy!

It certainly put everything into perspective for me. I've certainly had my challenges over the past few years, but reflecting on them, they were nothing compared to the battle my father would be facing against this disease. My father, my tall, great, gentle dad; he would be strong I knew it. I needed him to be; for me, my brothers, his grandsons, for my mum, and most of all for himself!

The greatest challenge for me was living so far away from my parents. I just wanted to be there, to give him a giant hug, and pass my strength through to him. I'm thousands of miles away, sitting in the United Kingdom, with him in Australia, and I felt helpless. Hearing the prognosis felt so much harder with such an immense distance between us. Whilst I always knew the choice I made many years ago to live in a different country would one day become difficult should such a situation arise, I had never really contemplated the reality of how I would feel when that day came. It suddenly felt like I couldn't breathe for the distance between me and my father.

My father has been so very proud of me through the years, sometimes unrealistically so. Nevertheless, that's what dads do! I called him this week after hearing the news. He told me not to worry, that it was '*just a hiccup*', and he went on to complain about the hospital food he was being fed, whilst he underwent more tests. That's my dad; always putting his best foot forward. Sometimes I wonder if he really is scared, and if he's trying to protect me from how he's really feeling. He must be scared. I certainly would be.

Dad was never one to openly share his personal emotions, his thoughts, or his fears. He would never hesitate to tell me, or any of the family that he loved us, but other than that, I never really knew if Dad was upset at something. He was always encouraging and barely griped about much at all. It did make it difficult to really understand him at times. He was quiet, reflective, always remaining optimistic for our benefit. Being so distanced from him, with our phone conversations or skype as the only connection, I certainly couldn't read him now. I felt I needed to be there, but to do what? Just wait? It's all about the wait right now. What next? The full prognosis and treatment plan would come in time, and whatever we needed to do, I want to help him fight against this disease.

My father is a war veteran, having served in Vietnam. He fought and survived one of the most terrible wars as an infantry soldier. In a battle with guerrilla warfare, my father and his comrades were often taken unawares. He experienced and witnessed things he could never explain to me, in a war that was cruel and treacherous; an experience that has continued to haunt him throughout the years. However, now he faces an entirely different battle altogether! The enemy here is entirely unseen, and it's dangerous. Nevertheless, I know my father and he is a brave soldier. He will go into combat for himself and his family. He is the ultimate war hero.

Distance aside; we will be there in battle with him, encouraging him and holding his hand every step of the way. I know my dad too well. We will prevail against this cruel enemy and live to fight another day!

Light from the Clouds

When my period arrived the next month, I was surprisingly okay. With my father's diagnosis, any thoughts around a potential pregnancy had taken a back seat. Strangely, in having a period, I knew my body had completed yet another full menstrual cycle and it gave me further reassurance that my body was recovering well from the Asherman's syndrome. In the midst of the bad news about my father, this was at least a small weight off my mind. Of course I still wanted to fall pregnant, and I certainly would have been overjoyed at a positive pregnancy test. However, my mind was on other things as I waited for updates on my father's health, hoping that the specialists and tests would produce something to provide us with an element of hope.

Naturally, we had every intention of continuing to try to have a baby. In a selfish way, I started to hope that a potential pregnancy might give my father the will to fight this horrid disease. I wanted him to see me become a mother, and to one day hold my baby; his grandchild. I feared now, that I was really running against time. It was all becoming a little overwhelming as I thought about my dad. My mind was in a constant blur, as I'd lay awake at night thinking about what the next few months would bring for him: tests, treatments, medication, more tests, worse? Yet despite this, the world keeps turning, and I have to get up each day and carry on without burdening my colleagues and friends with my woes. Work was relentless, and in some ways I suppose it gave me a daily distraction. It was at night that I'd lay awake, just thinking.

Perhaps it was a need for hope and good news, but suddenly I felt even more determined to succeed in our quest to get pregnant. We had two more months of trying before we would see the specialist again, and I thought it would be wonderful to present him with the good news of a successful conception. With two good cycles now, I felt confident that my body was ready for this – at last. I truly believed that it was my time to finally become a mother. Whilst it hasn't been an easy road, I had to believe that there is a rhyme and reason to Mother Nature's path, and this was my time! How did I know? I didn't, but I had to hope that I was right. If I didn't carry hope above everything else, I may as well have given up at that point altogether.

With that belief in mind, it became all about timing, waiting and dates once more. I earmarked my calendar to show when and where I would be over the next month, so that I could give myself the best chance of conception. On a daily basis, I was preparing myself, and counting the days before ovulation, and then after; right up to that exact date where I could take a pregnancy test. Pass or fail, this was a rite of passage I had re-entered, and strangely I was excited. In less than a month, I could be pregnant! Oh how I desperately wanted that to be true!

Just the thought brought butterflies to my stomach. For many women two months of trying is nothing, but for me it had been much longer than that. I was also very aware that getting pregnant was only my first hurdle. History had proven before that I could get pregnant. For me, the major milestone was hearing the first heartbeat. I knew it wouldn't be an easy road, and that I would need to control my anxiety up until that six or seven week scan. To be truthful, I wasn't sure how I would cope during those early weeks of pregnancy, and whether after all this time, I could even carry a baby to full term. However, after this long road, getting pregnant was the first step; the rest I would deal with as it arose. Right at this moment, I was allowing myself to become excited and celebrate my body's return to a degree of normality. I finally had the chance to try to conceive once again! That was something to celebrate on its own!

Perhaps giving myself a two-month time span to fall pregnant was a little ambitious, but most people will agree that I'm ambitious and I was willing to bet on those odds and remain positive. My body was showing all the signs that it was ready for this. I had the chance to *become pregnant* once more. That was something I had started to believe would never happen to us again. If I was able to conquer that hurdle, I was confident that I could clear the rest of them, and celebrate the New Year with a growing belly and the promise of a rainbow baby!

Glow in the Rain

As I reached the two-week wait once again, I was reminded why this process was so agonizingly frustrating. Just a week after ovulation, and with another week to go before my period was due, I started to feel a little cramping. Of course, my brain went into overdrive, and suddenly I had myself convinced that this must be implantation!

So firstly, it has been well over eighteen months since my last pregnancy, and I'm already over-thinking symptoms and setting myself into a frenzy of 'am I' or 'aren't I' pregnant delusions. I remembered all this from before, and although I was well aware of my past mistakes, somehow I couldn't stop myself from doing it again. I'm like an addict, I kept telling myself that I had this under control, but secretly, I was sneaking into the bathroom to check myself, giving myself false hopes, when I knew it was far too early to tell either way!

I had cramping which was light, and it coincided with the timing of what could be implantation, so I allowed myself a little bit of hope. Then, I was sure that my boobs felt more tender, perhaps another good sign. In my heart I wanted to believe this was happening, but I was also desperately trying to manage my expectations. I didn't want to get all my hopes up, only to have my period arrive at the end of the week. I kept telling myself that it wouldn't be terrible if we didn't get pregnant this month. Some couples wait several months before a positive test, and they hadn't experienced half the medical issues we had. However, I knew telling myself to remain patient wasn't going to work. I wanted it all now, of course.

It felt so frustrating, as I desperately willed everything to work in my favour. I'd find myself just touching my stomach at times, whispering a silent prayer to myself that this would be the month, that we would finally see that double line on a test. Whether it was in my head or real, as each day progressed, the common early pregnancy signs seemed to be telling me that perhaps we could be in luck this month. I dared to ask myself, *Could I be pregnant, just maybe?* I didn't say anything to anyone, as I didn't want to jinx my chances. At this stage, I didn't even tell my husband. I was definitely feeling more and more confident with each day leading up to my period due date. Something told me that this feeling was familiar, that I could be hopeful. The signs were all heading in the right direction. My period was due on the Friday and I had three days to go, but there were some definite tell-tale signs, mostly the obvious ones like bloating, cramping, tenderness and taste, yet I didn't dare do a test at this early stage.

On the Tuesday I was travelling for work overseas, so timing was perfect. I needed to stay distracted, and being in another country, busy all day in meetings, I knew I would barely have the time to think about the two-week wait until I returned home on the Friday evening. I deliberately chose not to pack a pregnancy test, knowing that I would give in to my paranoia and test early. Of course I cursed myself once I arrived in the hotel which was in the middle of nowhere, with no pharmacy in sight, should I change my mind. No turning back though, and if my period hadn't arrived by the time I returned home I wanted to ensure that my husband and I could do the test together.

Work conferences were always difficult during these times with ample coffee, interesting menu items, and of course, alcohol. Given my growing belief that we were pregnant I had to be careful, without raising any suspicions. I certainly wasn't going to risk this pregnancy if it was in fact there. I had suffered too many miscarriages to even tempt fate at this point in time.

By the Thursday, I was almost confident that this was our month, and I was looking forward to getting home the next day and seeing that positive pregnancy test. I opted to decline the group dinner that evening, the perfect excuse to avoid the sociality, including pre-dinner beverages, menu items I should avoid, and a late night. I was excited, and still very conscious of not taking my chances on anything so early if I was pregnant. Finally, the anxiety became too much to bear alone. I decided I had to share my thoughts with my husband, sending him a text just before the meeting closed. *'I am afraid of typing this just in case, but I think I might be pregnant'.* I knew that would get his attention, and sure enough my phone buzzed a few seconds later.

He was thrilled, and asked if I could get to a pharmacy. I texted back, telling him I wanted to wait until I was home the next day. I knew he would be excited too, but the realistic side of him also warned me not to get my hopes up. Too late, I thought.

With the meeting over, and my colleagues leaving the hotel for a night out, I was more than happy to order room service and call my husband. We spoke and he had already purchased some tests ready for my return the next day. The anticipation was immense, and I felt overjoyed that this could be finally happening. After such a long and tumultuous journey, this could be our time.

My stomach was still cramping, and I tried to recall how I had felt at this stage in my last pregnancies. The problem was that they were quite a while ago, and I struggled to recollect whether I had felt similar in my last pregnancies; it had been so long ago now I could barely remember.

As I watched television and enjoyed room service in the quiet of my small hotel room I relaxed, taking my time through the meal and looking forward to an early night. I started to get ready for bed early, looking forward to cosying up in the big hotel bed and finding something in English to watch as I fell asleep. It was when I was changing into my pyjamas in the bathroom, I saw that familiar stain on my underwear and realised that I had my period. Game over! There was no doubt at all in my mind; it had arrived one day early.

Disappointment flooded through me, as well as the realism that my hormones and cycle were probably sending me a variety of signals as they were returning to a regular menstrual pattern. Again, I had to tell myself that this wasn't completely bad news, but of course I felt betrayed by the signs my body had sent me all week. At least my cycles were regular, and perhaps I could have another chance next month. I had to find a positive in all this.

I phoned my husband immediately, and he was sympathetic and encouraging. We realised we were both ambitious to hope that it would happen so quickly. The signs were all good, and we knew that eventually I would get pregnant again; we just needed to show a little more patience, give it a little more time. I couldn't wait to get home tomorrow. I wanted to be with my husband, to just hold him and have him assure me that we would have our time eventually. In the meantime, I had to start mentally preparing myself for another month of trying. It was now almost a month before Christmas and we had three full cycles, and two months of actually trying. Already, I felt like we had been on this treadmill again for years.

Caught in a Whirlwind

When I started my fertility journey, I had always vowed to myself that I would never let it get in the way of my lifestyle. I didn't want to become the person so obsessed with my monthly cycle that I would cancel arrangements or suddenly drop everything because of time and ovulation windows. I had always looked to carry on with my life as normal, knowing that nothing was a sure thing, and prioritising my loved ones, family and friendships were also equally important. Life doesn't stop while you are waiting to fall pregnant.

However, slowly, as the years have progressed, I was feeling as though my fertility issues, the medical management of my condition, and now this desperate quest to get pregnant before Christmas had started to overrule my life in many ways. It was late November, and I needed to stop and check myself, as I had started to question my plans to spend the weekend away with a group of girlfriends. It was meant to be a pre-Christmas get-together, with gossip, food, wine and good laughs; yet at the same time it looked as though it would clash with my ovulation window. I suddenly hit a quandary, and I had no real excuse to get out of the weekend. Did I want to risk another month, when we had fought so hard to get to this place?

Again, I had to keep telling myself that there was no absolute guarantee we would even fall pregnant this month, and would I then be making the same decisions again next month for the same reason. Will these excuses just keep coming? How long do you put your life on hold for this? But, what if? That is, of course, a big 'if', but it is something. There is a voice inside my head that keeps reminding me that I need to give myself every opportunity.

It is especially relevant as I shift closer to my fortieth birthday, and my doctors continue to advise me that any chance of a successful pregnancy will continue to decrease each month. Therefore, each month that I'm not pregnant moves me further away from my dream of having a baby. Do I really want to risk it? I could be missing out on that successful pregnancy by de-prioritising everything around my social life.

So that is the selfish side of me speaking. But is it really selfish? Or is it sensible given everything we have been through?

I had to continue to remind myself that this wouldn't last forever; that there was only so much longer I could keep trying, as the path becomes narrower with each month that passes. Surely, I needed to keep up the pace now. And so, whilst I was on this path, surely I was entitled to make it my biggest priority? I realise that I'm justifying all this in my head, and yet I'm going against every principle I promised myself when starting this journey.

That realisation alone grounds me, and with all the hope in the world, I still have no control over my body. It would be wonderful to know for sure, that I could plan this, and know that by next Christmas we would finally have our baby with whom to celebrate the festive season. Yet the reality is that I could still be where I am today, or perhaps on a different journey altogether. Rightly or wrongly, I still had to be true to myself, focus on my personal well-being, and remain strong-willed and hopeful. If I can't 'live in the now' I would be essentially placing my entire life on hold for something that may only turn out to be a dream. Others may think differently, yet I have to stand by my own decision.

As I talked it over with my husband we agreed that this girls' weekend away may actually be better therapy for me personally, and it wouldn't necessarily count out our chances completely. It may actually prove to be a good distraction, to take the pressure off ourselves in the lead up to Christmas. We agreed that we weren't putting the brakes on trying, but that perhaps it might be beneficial for us to just enjoy the festive season without the anxiety of waiting and monitoring my menstrual cycle. We still had the appointment scheduled with my specialist early in the New Year, and even though we had only really tried for a pregnancy for two months so far, I felt we had a plan for exploring our future options with pregnancy, including the potential of undergoing a round of IVF.

Once the decision was made, I felt a little relieved, to be honest. I guess I hadn't realised how much I had been working myself up about this deadline to get pregnant by year end. My mind had become so over-ruled by this quest that it felt as though everything else had stopped around me, and I was becoming caught in a whirlwind of question marks.

On top of this, everything around me had been begun to feel a little heightened alongside this focus to get pregnant. With daily phone calls to my parents, I was anxious for regular updates on my father's prognosis. I knew it wasn't looking good for him, and even more so, I wondered if getting pregnant right now was even sensible. I needed to be prepared to jump on a flight home at any time. To top off things, work was nearing quarter and year-end, and therefore projects and deadlines were increasing, as I tried to keep my head above water. It wasn't until we had pushed our ambitions to get pregnant by Christmas aside that I realised how much pressure I had been placing on myself. I needed to get some air, find a release, and making that final decision gave us the excuse to just 'let go'.

Taking a step back also helped me rationalise my options, and getting home to Australia to visit my father was definitely a priority. My brother and his family had just returned from Australia, and whilst Dad was still in good spirits, he would be soon starting chemotherapy. Who knows how his body would react to this aggressive treatment. The next few months would certainly be an uphill battle for him, and with Christmas in just over a month, I needed to start thinking about my travel plans. I needed to see him, give him a hug, sooner rather than later.

Given his initial treatment schedule, I agreed with my mum that it would be best that I plan to get to Australia in February, following his first round of chemotherapy, and allowing him time to adapt and recover after his treatment schedule. Three months seemed such a long wait, but I hoped it would give my father something to look forward to. I also planned to return again on my own throughout the year as needed. I just needed my father to stay strong over the coming months; I wanted to be able to give him a hug, and to tell him that I loved him dearly, in person. Once we had booked our flights for February I felt as though a huge weight had lifted off my chest.

The whirlwind was still blowing a gale, but at least I could see my way through the next month or so, and I would let fate take its own course through the festive season and into the New Year.

A Seasonal Change

I love the festive season; it is honestly my favourite time of year. I had promised myself and my husband that I would focus on relaxing in the lead up to Christmas, and with everything else we had fully committed to throwing any thoughts of timing, pregnancies and the pressure out the window to just enjoy ourselves.

It may seem selfish and perhaps foolish, but I was now thinking that if we did keep actively trying, I would be potentially facing another Christmas and New Year with the worry of those first early weeks of pregnancy. My period was due a week before Christmas, and I was quite happy to shelve our plans and leave everything to chance. I wanted to start the New Year with a fresh start, hoping to assess my options once we had met with my specialist again. For many, this may seem a crazy plot, given my 'advancing age' and the time I have waited to get my cycle back. Why wouldn't I just keep trying, month after month, until we did get that positive result?

For me the answer is simple. My sanity!

It was the waiting, the build up and the anxiety that had started to get to me again. Also, if I was to fall pregnant again, I knew that those first few weeks would be incredibly stressful. Reaching our first milestone of six and half weeks would feel like an eternity! Then, if we did reach that, we would be entering further unknown territory, as we had never reached the point in our earlier pregnancies beyond a healthy heartbeat. I know my own anxieties well enough to understand that I would be on edge and paranoid throughout my entire pregnancy, right until I could finally hold my baby in my arms. I needed to allow myself some 'pause periods', allowing me to take my mind off the process of trying, and relax, letting life throw whatever it wants my way. If age is truly against me, this one-month won't make a world of difference.

Mother Nature had got me back to where I now had a fighting chance to get pregnant again. Of course I wasn't willing to waste it, but I also didn't want to risk it by sending myself insane with tests, trying, symptoms and other anxieties. Especially during a season which should be focused on family, friends and of course, festive cheer. It was more important that this year, I focus on my family, and put my own agenda and anxieties aside.

I won't deny that it has been difficult, and just picking up and starting festive celebrations with this at the back of my mind is challenging. At times, it felt as though something inside me was a little numb as I heard of babies being born all around me. Each Christmas I see my friends with their children, celebrating Christmas time, and I was still desperate to start this parenting journey.

I was reminded of this on a morning driving to work, as I listened to my normal breakfast radio station. My heart felt heavy as I listened to the excitement of young child callers telling the public of their Christmas wishes, decorating their trees and, of course, the anticipation of Santa's big arrival. It made me crave the children I have lost on this journey, and potentially the ones I may never have.

As a child, I was completely in love with Christmas; I would count down the days until Santa arrived, and I was truly swept up in the magic of the season. As an adult, I had dreamt of conjuring those feelings and experiences with my own children; hoping to one day watch the pure delight on their young faces on Christmas morning as they gathered around the Christmas tree to enjoy the true spirit of the day.

As a couple, we had now spent three Christmas Days as hopeful parents, and each year it became more difficult as we watched others celebrate the season with their growing families. Whilst I was still hopeful that next year we would finally celebrate the season as parents, the reality of whether that could actually be, still scared me. Perhaps our dreams of hiding presents, leaving notes for Santa, and filling a stocking full of toys for our own children may never come true.

So how would I cope this Christmas? I should just eat, drink and be merry - right? It did feel a little contrived.

For some reason, I had actually truly believed that we would be pregnant this Christmas, and that our plans entering the New Year would be focused on designing our nursery, maternity plans and the life-changing happiness that comes with starting a family. I did my calculations; if we did count this month out, by the time I reached my fortieth birthday, I still would not yet have become a mother.

For many who start to reach their forties, there are a lot of regrets. Well, I really only have the one!

Despite the true spirit of Christmas, this year I felt slightly empty, like there was a piece of me that was missing. Santa can't leave what I want under the tree; if only it were that easy.

Playing in Puddles

I am constantly amazed by how many women have faced various challenges with their fertility. Many continue to carry on with normal life, amidst IVF, tests, losses and the frustrations of aspiring to become a mother. We are often expected to keep going, keep working, keep carrying on with life, pretending that all is right in the world, when it really isn't.

This is my personal quandary right now. My career and my lifestyle still keep moving, and I can't just stop everything, knowing that we are hoping to start a family. What if we can *never* have children? There's no use placing life on hold for a 'what if'. Yet, I do find this concept hard at times. It's difficult to just ignore what's going on with my body and my emotions as I've hit each obstacle along the way. Also, can I keep going, and what sacrifices will I need to make to reach my goal?

Around me, at work, my colleagues know my

story, yet I assume that by now they believe we've possibly stopped actively trying. Why? Well, I guess it's an assumption, but it has also been over eighteen months since my last pregnancy. Mostly, I don't talk about our fertility issues at work unless I'm asked. Many have read my first memoir. Some will raise the subject, and if they want to know more, I'll enlighten them briefly about our journey. If I'm asked whether we are still trying, and at times I still get that question, I explain that the chapter is not closed, but I don't share more unless I'm probed, and mostly that doesn't happen. Perhaps it is out of respect, or maybe discomfort, but either way, I don't press the topic. Life goes on. I'm fully aware that people would most likely prefer not to listen to my woes of miscarriage and trying to conceive.

To be fair, do people really want to know *everything* about my fertility journey? For someone not living with it every day, it's not the most appealing topic of conversation. That doesn't offend me at all.

I generally just carry on, with my job and my hobbies, focusing on the task at hand, as there's no time to really wallow in my own self-pity. My work and my career have kept me going through all of this, helped me to maintain my sanity at the hardest of times. I've been incredibly fortunate to have the support of my colleagues where I've needed it, and at the end of the day, even if we had a child, I would still want to maintain my career in some way, shape or form.

My career and work has always been a backup plan for me. I knew that if we couldn't conceive and if we had to walk away from parenthood, I had the focus and ambition to take my career further. It wasn't my exact life plan, but the intensity with which I'd approach this would certainly be stronger if I was faced with a life without children. On the other hand, if we did have children, I had still always planned to return to work in some capacity. I understand that this subject forms one of those topical debates for women. Personally, I believe it's a personal choice, and fundamentally, it's about what makes you comfortable as a mother. I am who I am, and my child will want to know the real me as they grow and develop. That is important to me.

Change is inevitable in becoming a mother; I know that! I have pursued a career, and worked hard to reach my goals. Like my own mother, I had intended on finding a balance between both motherhood and my profession. I am my mother's daughter, and she was my inspiration growing up as she encouraged me to become a strong, independent woman. I would have hoped that one day, my own son or daughter would look to me with the same respect. But that is my path, and not everyone else's. If we were all the same life would be dull, and ultimately every child would grow up with the same mindset.

The path ahead still feels undefined to me, and even with the best-laid plans I am still waiting on our chance to demonstrate that this balance can truly work if I were to reach motherhood. In the meantime, I will continue to carry on with my life and work, knowing that it is at this point the one constant that I can control and rely on. Yet this begs the question; could I continue to cope at this pace, if we were to take the next step to IVF? Can I still strike this balance between work and my personal life? As my husband and I discuss this, and our pending appointment in the New Year, we find ourselves bouncing about with the pros and cons of undergoing the treatment.

Many have gone down the IVF road, I know, and the results have been successful. Only a few months ago I was solidly against IVF as an option, and yet we are re-opening the discussion. I'm told that my advanced age is now working against our chances of a successful pregnancy, or could even impact the chances of a baby being born with a disability. Having treatment, with a process of genetic screening would increase our chances of a successful, healthy pregnancy. However, my one question still remains: *Could we get there without the assistance of this process?*

With just a few weeks before Christmas I joined some friends for afternoon tea. One of them is a wonderful mother to a lovely little girl after successful IVF treatment. Perhaps it was the influence of champagne, but her description of the entire process for IVF sounded much more controlled than I had expected. The way she described her experience sounded so simple, and straightforward. She advocated the support and monitoring throughout, and made it sound much easier to manage than the unpredictability and guess work in each of my monthly cycles. *Was it really?* I had to ask myself.

It would certainly take the speculation out of the process, and being so closely monitored throughout every step would surely give me some assurance of the chances of success. From a timing perspective, it was a much more feasible option, particularly with my upcoming trip to Australia. I could plan any IVF schedule around those dates, taking away the unpredictability that we were forced to face with trying naturally. But what if it doesn't work on the first round? Do we give up and just walk away from it all? Can we really only do one IVF cycle?

Then there are the appointments, scans, hospital treatments. How does this work with a busy career? Up until this point in time I had maintained that balance so well, but I wasn't sure how my body would react to a new set of treatments, and whether it was truly possible to just 'carry on as normal' once more. I am committed to exploring the options, but with so many questions this was an entirely new territory for me. The doubts I had a few months back had certainly not disappeared. The thought of pumping a myriad of drugs and stimulants through my body still concerns me. On top of this, I am worried about the emotional, physical and financial effect it will have on us as a couple. We have stayed strong through everything so far, but what if this is too much for us. Will we cope? Can we survive more pain?

I am positive that many couples like me must have the same fears and doubts. At the same time, there is a small glimmer of hope that resides inside me, and that is what keeps me looking for new opportunities to realise my dream of being a mother one day. We've set the appointment for early January, with no firm commitments. However, it is another option to consider, and we will decide then if it's the path we take, and if so what our limits will be on that journey. We have to have limits, but at this point in time, I don't have the answers, and that's okay.

So let's just explore it, and see what happens next!

The Morning Dew

I have always envied those women who 'accidently' fell pregnant just as they stopped trying. I always wondered whether they actually did stop, or perhaps they just told everyone they had to avoid the questions and raised eyebrows. Perhaps I'm just cynical, but I had tried desperately over the years to put this quest out of my mind, and yet it never truly disappeared.

Even this month! Whilst we weren't trying, and actually I wasn't monitoring my cycle at all, I would always think about it. The difference is that this month, we barely 'actively' pursued a pregnancy (if you know what I mean). Mostly because our pre-Christmas social events were conflicting with any opportunity for us to 'try to get pregnant' and I had put the calendar away, as we had agreed.

Yet I knew if I told people we weren't trying, they would still doubt it. Who wouldn't after all we'd been through? I am constantly aware that people watch me and my behaviour regularly, watching my every move, and quietly observing my habits; yet most will avoid asking me whether we are having any luck on our quest to become pregnant. Whilst we don't often talk about it, I know that at times people will assume and sometimes that feels worse. It's the elephant in the room in many conversations; so much so that I make it clear on first meetings with friends I have not seen for a while that we are not yet pregnant. It is easier somehow to simply clear the air upfront, avoid any misunderstandings, and just be myself without any pretence.

At times, when I look at the reality, I feel a little frustrated. It's now been eighteen months since my last pregnancy. This has been the longest period I've experienced between pregnancies (having had four pregnancies within a two-year period previously), and it had become disheartening. Since my last miscarriage, I've undergone a myriad of medical appointments, investigations, different drugs and procedures, all in the hope that it would get us back to at least a pregnancy to start with. Whilst we have unofficially agreed to take a break over this festive season, these thoughts are never really far from my mind. It's a quest that is not yet over for me, and like with any break, I'm conscious there is always a start and an end.

We had planned our Christmas Day to be spent with my brother, his wife and two young boys. I was looking forward to spending the day in our own home with the chaos of Santa's arrival, and enjoying the joy of Christmas Day seen through the eyes of a five and almost two year old. It will certainly bring the festive spirit into our celebrations! I've been looking forward to ensuring their day is as magical as the ones I had enjoyed as a young girl.

The New Year would bring new opportunities for decisions about our future as potential parents; however, for now, both my husband and I were happy to just enjoy ourselves. The more we considered it, the more we were contemplating IVF as an option to pursue, even if it meant waiting until after our return from Australia. Our consultation, which was booked for the week after New Year's Day, would hopefully answer the questions we needed to ask to help guide us.

At our last appointment, my specialist had expressed a strong preference for us to consider IVF, emphasising that a woman my age would face much better odds with a successful and controlled pregnancy. His words kept circling around me as we faced the year-end. I didn't want to spend more months trying, waiting and predicting, or even worse, failing! With all the advancements in medical interventions and everything we've been through so far, surely IVF was the best option for a successful, full-term pregnancy. It was a big and costly decision, and despite our frequent yo-yoing around the subject, I felt that as a couple, we were starting to warm to the idea, at least as a strong consideration.

So, what happens when you suddenly find yourself pregnant?

It was the Monday and Christmas was the coming Friday. Amidst the last minute present buying and catching up with friends, I suddenly realised that my period was due yesterday. I hadn't thought too much about it as my stomach had been cramping over the past few days and I was expecting the arrival of my menstrual cycle, but it never came. I hadn't really thought to test; I just assumed it was my body playing tricks on my once more. But, late this afternoon, I had a thought that perhaps I should just pee on that stick to find out either way. I doubted it would turn out positive, but I had a spare pregnancy test in our bathroom cabinet, and on a whim, I did the test. As I sat there, it was at first what I had expected. There was one strong control line and nothing more. Then, as I washed my hands and picked up the test again, about to throw it away, I looked again. I squinted, thinking it was perhaps my eyes playing tricks, but I could have sworn there was a faint second line beginning to appear. It was barely visible, but I was sure I could see it. I sat in that bathroom for a long while, waiting for the test to dry, trying to control my emotions, should this be just a mind trick. It was there, a light pink line! *I couldn't be, could I?*

I quickly went through the cabinet, pulling out a digital test this time. Yes, I carried plenty of spare tests for such emergencies. A girl can never be too prepared. However, my bladder was empty, and I had to wait. I was too afraid at this stage to even admit that there was the possibility. The thought of being pregnant seemed inconceivable. This month had been such a random and relaxed month; I honestly couldn't remember how it could be possible. Drinking down glassfuls of water, I tried desperately to think about dates and possibilities. Giving myself plenty of time, I went back to the bathroom almost two hours later.

Lo and behold it came through, *'Pregnant 1-2'*! I was completely in shock. I couldn't believe it, yet the small words on the little black screen were staring right back at me.

I was pregnant!

I took the test downstairs. My husband was in the lounge watching television. I jumped on the sofa next to him, waving the stick in his face.

"What?" he asked dumbfounded. "How?"

"I have no idea!" I said grinning stupidly; it was suddenly really dawning on me. My smile became an excited giggle. "My period was due yesterday, and when it didn't come..." I stopped, it just seemed so unimaginable but incredibly delightful. Suddenly, we had a completely new angle on our situation.

It was still very early days. I was only four weeks pregnant. Suddenly, all of our declarations about enjoying Christmas and New Years and thinking about our parental plans in January were now out the window. Who cares! I was pregnant! Getting pregnant at all was a major milestone given our history. Even better, this was a natural pregnancy. The pregnancy I was told I could never really achieve again, and yet, we did it! I couldn't have been happier. I still had to control my emotions, and at only four weeks in, I was well aware that we had a long road ahead, and getting to that first heartbeat at six or seven weeks was our first significant step. In those first few minutes of discovering I was pregnant, all those feelings started to frighten me once more. I desperately hoped that this time I would make it past six weeks, and whilst I was overjoyed, I was also terrified.

"This is good news," my husband said gently, staring into my eyes, and reading my thoughts. I nodded unconvincingly. I had gone from over the moon, elated, to suddenly petrified. "One step at a time," he said reassuringly, pulling me to him and holding me tight. I smiled again. It had happened. It was what we had hoped for all along, and I couldn't let my fears overrule this amazing moment. *We were pregnant at last!*

So Merry Christmas to me! Perhaps Santa really was listening this year?

A Shift in the Storm

Later that evening I started working out my dates, and I realised with even more surprise that this baby was due exactly on my fortieth birthday. Surely this was a positive sign?

Any woman who has been through any kind of loss, frustration or waiting, will appreciate that finally getting that positive pregnancy test is somewhat bittersweet. On one end, I couldn't be happier; yet given my past, I felt that there was a constant shadow threatening my happiness. That night I went to bed holding my stomach, knowing that there was a little life forming in there, and willing it to be strong and healthy.

It was as though that dark shadow was determined not to let me get ahead of myself as I woke the next morning. Perhaps I had expected something to happen from the very start, and my pessimism had influenced my fate. As soon as went to the bathroom I knew something was wrong before I even checked. The cramping I had felt for the past two days felt stronger, and when I checked my underwear, there was blood.

"Shit!" I cried.

"What's wrong?" my husband called through the closed door. Tears sprung from my eyes; it was happening again.

"I'm bleeding," I called back miserably, knowing what this meant. I tried to look at the bright side of the situation. I had fallen pregnant, and naturally. Therefore, we could get here again, right? Only a day in, I hadn't built up too many expectations, and I had to be glad that it was perhaps over with quickly. My mind raced through a number of justifications, trying to appease the growing ache in my heart.

This wasn't like my other miscarriages. It was very early, and I had to think of the positives, despite the disappointment. I had started to doubt our ability to ever fall pregnant again, and yet I had beaten the odds. My husband was standing on the other side of the door when I finally opened it and he held his arms out to hold me. His eyes told me the same thing; it was disappointing but still positive. We got pregnant in the first place! If we could get to this place once (in only three months) we could make it here again. We just had to make the pregnancy stick.

As soon as I had rationalised these thoughts, it didn't feel as devastating. Perhaps after all this time, my emotions are more controlled, or perhaps I am just used to experiencing the loss; but I felt much calmer about the fact that this pregnancy had come and gone. My husband kept checking on me all morning, and I had to keep reassuring him that I was actually okay.

I kept checking myself throughout the day, and the bleeding wasn't heavy, but it was enough to tell me that this was not a good sign. Christmas was three days away, and I still had a lot to organise beforehand. At least I could keep my mind occupied I thought, as I assured my husband that I would be okay. We both agreed to treat this as a positive experience, and focus on keeping our festive spirit alive.

That same day, I had planned to meet a good friend for lunch in London, and I was determined not to let this setback get to me. Taking the train into Euston station I was looking forward to a good pre-Christmas catch up. I did confide in her about what happened, and she was terrible disappointed for me, knowing exactly what we had been through to date. At twenty weeks pregnant herself, she knew too well the anxiety of those early weeks of pregnancy. By this stage though, I had written my pregnancy off, and told my friend that I had to see the positive in the situation. This pregnancy had given me hope. This storm was passing; I was sure of it. I was content to ride out this bad weather, and focus my sights on a bright new year ahead. I would get pregnant again!

Taste of Rain

I really am not meant to have it easy throughout this process. Perhaps, somewhere, someone is truly testing me. I had convinced myself it was all over, and hadn't given the pregnancy much more thought over the next day or so. I had to be realistic. Those cramps were bad, and with the bleeding on top of that at such an early stage, it was not a good sign. I didn't bother going to a doctor, as they couldn't have done anything at just over four weeks. I had to wait it out.

When the cramps and bleeding finally subsided, I joked with my husband that we should top up the champagne order on our Christmas food order. I had diagnosed myself as having a chemical pregnancy – a miscarriage that occurs so early on that it only ever shows a positive pregnancy test, but disappears quickly after. It was the only thing that made sense. Never before had I had a positive test, and then had bleeding so quickly. My pregnancy was gone before I had even had a chance to really appreciate it. However, I was surprisingly okay with that. Perhaps because it was so early, or because I hadn't expected to even be pregnant. In many ways, I felt fortunate to have found out early, rather than wait weeks (like in my prior pregnancies) to find out that the pregnancy hadn't survived.

It was Christmas Eve, and I was busily preparing for my brother and his family to arrive, when I started to question whether my diagnosis was actually correct. I felt strange. Something, perhaps a gut feel, told me that perhaps I should do another test, just to check. After all, I wanted to indulge on Christmas Day with lots of food and wine; but I needed to be sure that this pregnancy was declining for sure. I told myself I was being silly, giving myself false hope, and it was my mind simply playing tricks on me. Regardless, I went to the pharmacy and picked up another set of pregnancy tests. Better safe than sorry, right?

In my view, if this pregnancy was disappearing, there would be no progression in the results. The line would be fainter; and the digital test would show 'not pregnant' or remain where it was on that first test I did on the Monday, displaying only '1-2 weeks'. When I did the first test, there were two lines again. *No surprise*, I told myself, *the pregnancy hormone would perhaps still be in my body*. So, I did the second test with the digital display.

I felt irrational and silly as I watched the little timer blink, becoming impatient with myself for being so delusional. It kept blinking, and predicting the result I took the pending test downstairs to my husband and asked him to watch it for me. I kept rationalising that I needed the peace of mind, and I could tell my husband thought that the test was unnecessary as well.

When it finally flashed up, we both stared at each other in shock. First the word 'Pregnant' appeared, and we continued to wait. The little timer was still blinking. It was taking much longer than last time. Our eyes were both glued to the little screen for what seemed an eternity. I stood up, aggravated at the wait. I knew for sure the pregnancy hormones were still swimming around in my body, but this was torture. Finally, the blinker stopped, and the second line appeared: '2-3 weeks'.

"Holy crap!" I said disbelievingly.

"What does this mean?" My husband looked at me.

"I think we can say that I'm still pregnant." I shook my head. "I don't understand, though... That cramping and the bleeding. I was so sure that was it."

My husband nodded, still looking at the test in his hands. There was no doubt, whatever had happened a few days ago, hadn't stopped this pregnancy from progressing. I was still pregnant, and tomorrow was Christmas Day.

We told my brother and his wife, as of course, we agreed to remain safe over Christmas, with me steering clear of alcohol, caffeine and any other unsafe foods. I was still nervous, as it felt like we were giving ourselves false hope, but what else could we do? *How could this honestly be?* I kept asking myself. I had never had a bleed like this before so early in pregnancy, and even then, I had never reached past the first seven weeks. I was still sure this wasn't going to last.

Christmas Day was fun, and I enjoyed myself, letting myself accept this pregnancy for what it was: a blessing. Whether it stayed or went, we were pregnant and it was Christmas. Santa arrived with lots of gifts for my nephews, and we were quickly enveloped into the spirit and mayhem of Christmas day with two young excitable boys.

We went to a friend's house party on Boxing Day, and again I remained calm and low key throughout the celebrations. It was hard to truly celebrate, with this irrational fear of loss still looming over me. I wanted to protect my emotions, and it was too early to share my news. With each day progressing, I was afraid of giving myself more hope, when I knew that nothing was guaranteed. As we arrived home in the evening, I started to experience more cramping. My fears re-emerged, as I lay in bed that night, my stomach contracting the same way it had just under a week ago. Not a good sign.

During the night, I woke in pain, and when I went to the bathroom I found even more blood. Seriously, when was I going to get a break? I felt cheated, and I now just wanted this over with. It was as though a cruel joke was being played at my expense as this was being dragged out. The next morning the bleeding had mostly ceased, but the cramping was still strong. It was a bank holiday and everything would be closed, and this wasn't considered an emergency, so I had no option but to lie in bed, and rest.

Then, as if that wasn't enough, I called my mum, to give her an update. Always positive, my mum wanted to remain hopeful, but I could even hear her hesitation when she offered me sympathy. She also gave me some difficult news from her end. Something had happened with Dad over the past twenty-four hours. Like me, there was not much she could do during the holidays, but she said he wasn't himself and seemed to get confused very quickly. Mum feared that the cancer had spread to his brain, as he couldn't even pick up a spoon at the dinner table. She had called the emergency doctors, who had advised that she should call the specialist during office hours the next day.

My situation felt so menial compared to my dad's, and my anxiety seemed to quadruple as I hung up the phone. I wanted to scream and punch something, as my stomach seized again. How could I share another loss with my family when they were dealing with such an enormous situation themselves? I felt selfish and sorry for myself.

The cramps subsided again by the following day, and I reconciled with myself that this pregnancy was certainly doomed. Regardless, I decided to go to the doctor. Since my traumatic encounter with the doctor months earlier, I had re-registered with a new surgery; however, I had yet to meet my new doctor. What an introduction! I wanted desperately to avoid tests and examinations again, as the memories of past pregnancies and their losses came flooding back. It all felt like a bout of déjà vu! Alas, however, it had to be done.

The doctor was very empathetic, as I told him my history, and the events of the past week. I already knew that it was too early for a scan, but he suggested a blood test to see if my levels were where they should be for a pregnancy that would be just on five weeks. The results would be returned to me within twenty-four hours. At the same time, my father was referred to his own specialist for further tests and a CT scan, but he wouldn't know the results until after the New Year. All my expectations of a great start to the year were starting to fall away quickly. I felt utterly miserable on all ends, and I wanted to hide myself away from the world and wallow in my own pity. It wasn't fair.

When after twenty-four hours, I called for my own blood test results, the doctor advised that the count was quite good, but he still could not give me an absolute conclusion on the viability of this pregnancy. Whilst I still showed to be pregnant, that could be my body stubbornly holding onto the hormones. His only advice was to wait until six weeks to be scanned. Hesitantly, I agreed, and he booked an appointment with the early pregnancy unit for the following Tuesday when they re-opened. I dreaded that place with a vengeance. All my past memories of failed pregnancies had come from that small scanning room in the local hospital. Many of those experiences had left me upset, frustrated and unsupported. I really didn't want to go back there, and I felt that I was walking into further bad news by agreeing to the appointment.

On the morning of New Year's Eve, I felt less like celebrating, and more like hiding. My mother hadn't any further news on my dad, but at least his condition hadn't worsened. My cramps had completely disappeared, but I felt like rubbish, as I had also contracted a cold. If you could throw anything else at me I think I would have imploded. Still fearing that I was pregnant, I avoided taking any cold and flu medication, which made me even more miserable. This constant yo-yo was starting to wear thin. I still had a remaining digital test, and stupidly decided I should just use it up. Secretly and sadly, I hoped it would go backwards and just put me out of this misery. I had now completely convinced myself that this pregnancy was doomed one way or another, and I just wanted the worst of it over with. This time, when the test flashed its result, I felt physically sick. The little screen showed, 'Pregnant, 3+' and confirmed that the hormones were continuing to increase in my body. I really didn't know how I could interpret what was happening. I was getting so many mixed signals from this pregnancy, and whilst I was, of course, grateful the test came out with something to hope for, I was still extremely confused.

With the time zone differences between Britain and Australia, I couldn't even update my mum until the evening. She was, of course, worrying about my dad, as well as worrying about me. I didn't want to add to her woes, so I sent a cheerful note to her when I knew she would be awake with the latest test result.

You have a little fighter in there. Her text responded to me encouragingly. I desperately wanted to believe her but I just couldn't. There was still this nagging shadow sitting over my head, and we had been here before. I had become such a pessimist, and this last week or so certainly hadn't helped my mindset.

I hope so, I responded back. I really hoped that the 'little fighter' inside of me would fight hard; I hoped that he or she could even encourage my father to fight harder. With my due date as my fortieth birthday and my father's prognosis, could this pregnancy be a sign of fate? Could the promise of a new life keep everyone else's hope alive?

This year, I refused to make any new year's resolutions, but I did make a wish. I wished that by some miracle, this pregnancy would push through all these obstacles, and I would return to Australia in February at just over thirteen weeks pregnant and moving into my second trimester. I felt a little foolish pinning my hopes on something that had not looked positive to date, but I had to go into the New Year with a positive outlook. I had to focus on staying hopeful.

We drove home that night. I, of course, hadn't been drinking, and I wanted my own bed so that I could sleep in and rest the next day. Full of cold, feeling miserable and just not in the mood to really celebrate into the early hours of the morning, my husband and I left the party we had attended. He was a little tipsy, and I was glad he had enjoyed himself. I felt bad for leaving just after midnight, but he assured me that going home to our own bed was the right thing to do. He understood.

On the drive home we spoke. I really didn't want to go to the local hospital for that scan on Tuesday. I felt so negative about my past experiences there, and even though we had many signs telling me that this pregnancy was at risk, I still couldn't face hearing bad news again in that same place.

"When will you be six weeks?" my husband asked.

"In two days," I replied, which would be the Monday. "We could pay for a private scan," I suggested tentatively. I knew we didn't have to spend the money, especially as the NHS scan was already booked.

"If it makes you feel better, I'm happy to book the private scan," my husband agreed.

I did wonder if the little bit of drink in him make him more affable, but I was grateful all the same for his support. It was late, I was tired, and when we arrived home, I went straight to bed. I would find a private, local ultrasound clinic in the morning and make the appointment as agreed.

To this day, none of my past four pregnancies have ever made it beyond six weeks and four days' gestation, and I have always had a slow heartbeat or none at all. Getting past that hurdle would be absolutely amazing. I didn't want to build up my hopes, but an early scan would at least give me the reassurance we needed that perhaps (just perhaps) this pregnancy was growing. Did I dare to let myself even believe that was a possibility?

Temperature Check

I openly admit that I'm not a patient person. However, the first few weeks of any woman's pregnancy surely tests the boundaries of tolerance. Each day is one step forward, but as many women will advocate, it is all about getting through that first trimester.

For me, it is about getting to that first heartbeat. At this early stage, it's all I can focus on. On New Year's Day I stayed in bed, trying desperately to recover from this cold, but only able to drink orange juice and take Paracetamol (the only pain killer I was allowed) sporadically. I was miserable. Not just because of the cold, but because again I was so sure that I would be facing another pregnancy loss. I couldn't see how this pregnancy would last through what I'd been through in the last week or so. I had to prepare myself, and I wouldn't let myself get my hopes up, yet still I knew I needed to have the scan, to confirm what I already knew.

Rarely do I allow myself a full day in bed, but today I gave myself the exception. At least the bleeding and cramping had stopped, but as I went into fits of coughing and sneezing, I felt that none of it could be good for an early pregnancy. I found a few local private ultrasound places online, and one in particular that would be open the next day, which was a Saturday. At least I could call them and book an appointment. I expected they would be busy at this time of the year, and assumed that I wouldn't get an appointment until the following week. I was five weeks and five days pregnant, and well aware that it was unlikely to even detect a heartbeat until over six weeks. All of my past pregnancies had dated at least a week behind my actual dates, so it was better to wait a little longer, I consoled myself.

I didn't sleep much that night as thoughts ran around my head, with the anticipation of getting this appointment scheduled and getting some news either way. When I did phone first thing the next morning, I was surprised when the receptionist advised that an appointment was available at three o'clock that afternoon. It was pure luck, but of course I jumped on it. She asked my dates, and warned me that at five weeks, six days, there wouldn't be a heartbeat, and not much to see (if anything). I acknowledged her warning, telling her that I just wanted to know if the pregnancy was progressing, and that I would keep my expectations limited. Essentially, all I wanted to know was how far I was dating. I knew in advance that if the scan shows a pregnancy dating at around five weeks when I should almost be six, it would confirm my suspicions – that another miscarriage was imminent.

In my mind, I knew I should have waited to schedule this appointment for at least a few days later, but I didn't care. I needed to know now, and if I had to book a follow up scan in a week I knew I would do that, too.

I was nervous as we sat in the waiting room. The clinic was very friendly, much different from the public system, and the environment felt different, which helped a little. However, I couldn't help but start to work myself up as we waited to be called in.

When we did go in, the woman was very kind. She explained that I was having a *very* early scan, but that, hopefully, she should be able to see something to give us an indication of our dates. That's all I wanted. There was a large screen in front of both of us, so that we could see exactly what she was seeing. I saw the small blob immediately; there was definitely still a pregnancy. She asked me to wait whilst she did some measurements. As I expected, it was too early yet to detect the heartbeat, but to our wonderful surprise the pregnancy was at exactly five weeks and six days measuring a minute 2.9 millimetres. She explained she could see a small gestational sac and a yolk sac and that all was looking on the right track. I can't explain the sudden flow of emotions that ran through me as she told me this!

This was the first time ever that we had a scan dating on schedule. Yet I was still completely confused about what had been happening over the past week. She wasn't a doctor and couldn't give me any advice, but suggested that it may have been a form of implantation. It was the only explanation that seemed to make sense, and I certainly wasn't going to question it. I had fully expected to walk away from the scan with bad news, but now I could hardly hold in my excitement.

The apprehension didn't completely disappear of course, but I was reassured by the scan results, and the little blob we had seen on that monitor encouraged me. I could only keep hoping that we would get to a healthy heartbeat. I kept the appointment with my specialist for early January. I knew that it would be a different consultation to the one we had originally planned. We wouldn't be talking about IVF now. However, I knew he would be able to scan me at that appointment and I would be well over six weeks pregnant, and hopefully we would get our wish – a healthy pregnancy and a strong beating heart! Could I actually hope that this pregnancy – number five – would be our rainbow baby?

Distant Clouds

Despite our wonderful news, back home in Australia, the news wasn't as positive for my father. They had found small cancer cells in his brain, and he had suffered a series of small strokes just before the New Year. It explained his delirium, but it wasn't good news as far as his prognosis. He was now battling both lung cancer and brain cancer.

The good news was that he was feeling better, less cloudy, and starting to return to his old self. However, I felt for my mum who was desperately working through hospital staff and specialists, trying to get more answers about the progress of his cancer. The specialist could only advise her that it was advancing, that any treatment would not cure but only prevent its aggressive advancement. It was recommended that he ceased further chemotherapy treatment and started a round of radium on his brain. The main focus was to prevent further strokes, which were affecting my father's mental state.

The reality of my early pregnancy and the expectations of the coming months seemed to take a back seat with this news. My youngest brother was in Brisbane, and he was of course there to support my parents, but it still felt as though I was letting them down by not being there. What could I do? I couldn't exactly stop work, leave my house and home, and move back to Australia?

It really wasn't that simple. Especially now with a baby on the way. Finally I had what I wanted, a growing pregnancy. Yet there was a part of me that felt guilty, knowing that this pregnancy would rule the next several months of my life; that is if it continued to grow.

I started to fear what would be. What if I did have a successful pregnancy, but something happened to Dad in my later stages? Would I be able to get home in an emergency? How would I feel if I couldn't be there when things became critical?

It was my mum who put my anxieties in order when I spoke to her of my worries. She assured me that my dad was literally over the moon with the news of my pregnancy.

"He couldn't be happier for you!" She said to me encouragingly. "He wants to see your baby and he told me he won't give up." Mum's words brought tears to my eyes. Just the thought of my dad not being able to see my baby was unthinkable. He had to make it.

"Tell him to at least hold on until I can get there in nine weeks." I said sadly. I didn't know if I was being pessimistic or not, but I couldn't be sure. Nine weeks wasn't a long time, but right now, it felt like a lifetime.

"He'll be here." Mum said softly. "He wouldn't miss it for the world." Somehow, I knew she was right.

Ray of Light

I think my specialist almost fell off his chair when we arrived at our appointment. I was seven weeks exactly at our appointment, and when we told him our news, he was in shock. Like us, he didn't expect us to be pregnant at this meeting, but also, he emphasised that getting pregnant naturally within the first three months of trying was a great achievement.

He didn't keep me waiting, showing me straight to his ultrasound room, and assuring me that all signs so far were good. *At seven weeks there should be a heartbeat*, I told myself, hoping that we would get good news. He also had a monitor on display, so again I could watch what he was seeing, and straight away I saw our little blob.

"You have a heartbeat!" the specialist said confidently.

"Really?" I asked disbelievingly. I could barely breathe. "Is it a good heartbeat?" I quickly added.

"Yes, it's a good strong heartbeat," he said reassuringly.

I smiled as the wave of relief swept over me. I looked at my husband who squeezed my shoulders, and we smiled at each other.

The specialist started moving his cursor around the screen, taking measurements. "You are measuring at six weeks and six days," he said matter-of-factly. "At this early stage we are talking the difference of sub-millimetres, but it's all looking good in there so far."

"And the heartbeat is strong?" I asked again. I must have sounded foolish, but I honestly couldn't believe it.

"Yes," he laughed at me. "Getting to a healthy heartbeat is the first significant milestone, ninety percent of pregnancies survive to full term once we've seen that. Still, I suggest another scan in just over a week given your history."

I nodded eagerly. I was grinning like a Cheshire cat. We had never reached this stage in any pregnancy before, and I couldn't believe that we would be going home with a little scan picture and good news! I texted my mum immediately, even though it was some ungodly hour in Australia, I knew she would be waiting in anticipation for the results of our scan today. *'We have a healthy heartbeat!'* I sent. Immediately my phone buzzed back. It must be three in the morning there, and her sleepy but excited reply was, '*Excellent news xxx*'.

For the first time in weeks, I actually relaxed. We still had a very long road ahead, I knew that, but this milestone was significant given our history. As we boarded our train back home, I looked at my husband, who hadn't really spoken.

"What's wrong?" I asked cautiously.

"It's really happening," he said, his eyes quite wide with shock. It surprised me to see his reaction. He had always remained so positive through everything in this pregnancy, reassuring me to stay positive. What I realised was that he too had been surprised by today's results. I smiled at him proudly. We might actually be parents in around eight months' time. It felt surreal. "I guess we should start planning..." he suggested cautiously.

"Let's wait," I responded. This was a positive move forward, but I knew that there were still risks. "I just want to get to the first trimester," I said to him, as I held his hand. He nodded. I was content enough to hold the little scan photo of my baby blob in my hand, and celebrate the fact that the growing life inside of me had a strong beating heart. It was a blessing to even have made it this far.

My specialist had prescribed me daily injections of blood thinners, and also a progesterone suppository, which I'd need to take until fourteen weeks. All of these things were to help my pregnancy keep growing healthily. I didn't care. I was glad to have the support of modern medicine, and I could only hope that it would help our little baby to keep meeting its milestones. He also advised that we should undergo certain tests at around ten weeks to test for chromosomal and other disabilities. All were precautions, which kept reminding me that this road was not going to get any easier. Nonetheless, I was prepared to face anything to fight for this little life inside me. The destination will be well worth the discomfort of the journey.

I booked myself back into the private ultrasound clinic that we had first visited at just over eight weeks. I was still avoiding the public system at this stage, and I was much more comfortable with the service of the clinic, even if we had to pay for it ourselves. Even though the last scan was positive, within the week, I was worrying again. I kept telling myself I had nothing to be negative about now. There had been no more cramps or bleeding, and all my physical signs were positive. Yet, I kept feeling hesitant. *Could it be too good to be true*, I wondered. I also needed to protect my heart and my emotions, should this suddenly be taken away from me at any moment. Building up my hopes could only set me up to fall harder if the pregnancy did fail.

We were just over eight weeks at this third scan, and the results dated again on schedule. That little fighter in my belly was growing well, and this time, it looked more like a blobby tadpole. The consultant played the heartbeat for us to hear, and the sound was music to my ears. Sounding like a train, the heart was strong and fast, exactly as it should be. I looked over to my husband who had been watching the monitor intently. *It was unbelievable*, I thought to myself, smiling. This is what it should have felt like those other four times; this is what we had missed out on. The measurements were eight weeks and two days, and the little blob was still tiny at just under two centimetres. I couldn't imagine that something so small inside me had so much capacity to draw such happiness, but it did!

We agreed to get a further scan at ten weeks, as well as an early blood test, which would screen us for any disabilities such as Downs Syndrome. Each of these conditions has their own significant risks on the growth of my pregnancy. I'm advised that the likelihood of having a baby with chromosomal abnormalities is higher, given I'm turning forty this year, as a direct result of the quality and age of my eggs. Another obstacle we were forced to face on this difficult and long journey.

I wanted, therefore, to find out as early as possible if there would be any concerns with my baby, especially as I was very aware of the greater risk of such conditions with my age. Any decision that we'd have to make now would be extremely difficult; I knew that. I was starting to bond with my pregnancy, allowing myself to dream about what could be when he or she is born. I was starting to let myself believe that I would be a mother in a matter of several months. Each day forward was going to make it harder and harder if something were to go wrong. The scans were also important for me, as they were my only opportunity at this early stage to reassure myself that the pregnancy was okay. The time between these scans was excruciating and all my anxieties would begin to resurface as each date grew nearer.

I promised myself never to take anything for granted in this pregnancy, knowing that each day forward is a blessing, and should we reach full term with a healthy baby, it will all be worth the struggle and this emotional roller coaster that I've been riding for years now. One step at a time.

Dawn of a New Day

The first trimester is certainly a difficult time. We had told only a very select few people about our pregnancy. My parents of course; I needed my dad to know, it was only fair, and I wanted him to hear my news; I was hoping it may give him something positive to look forward to. We also told my brother and his wife, my mother-in-law, a few very close friends and my direct manager at work. Many couples keep absolute silence due to the uncertainty of the first trimester. However, given our history, and the need to frequently visit doctors, specialists and clinics, we wanted to trust a few people to support us through this anxious time. My workplace has also seen the worst of my history with past pregnancies, and it was only fair to ensure that they were aware of my current situation. The support I've received from work has been unwavering, and of course it didn't change with this news. I felt relieved to have disclosed the news, and with start of the year events and meetings, it was helpful to have an ally when I couldn't uphold some of those commitments.

For the rest, keeping the pregnancy a secret is almost like a full time job itself. With my openness on the subject, there were many people who have been watching my habits, knowing of our desire to become parents. Consequently, I decided to avoid some social events allowing me to escape the questions, and maintain my composure throughout this very anxious time. Those who knew were the people I wanted to talk to, if I felt my anxieties suddenly taking over my rational thinking. Outside of that, I wanted to carry on, hoping that in a few short weeks I would be able to proudly declare my pregnancy openly as it reached the second trimester.

At ten weeks and one day we arrived for the scan and the tests. Despite my imaginings of sudden bad news, we were once again proven wrong as our baby dated ten weeks and four days, still with a strong, healthy heartbeat, and this time looking a little more like a baby with a big head and a round little body with what looked like legs forming. It was amazing to watch the progress over the four scans, as that early tiny blob started to take shape.

We were then taken to another consulting room, where the blood test was to be done. The woman was kind, explaining that the test would take approximately five days for the results to come through, and that they would call me directly as soon as they received them. Regardless of the scans, this was particularly scary. What would we do if the results showed a serious disability? With some disabilities the pregnancy wouldn't survive, regardless. At this stage, my body still hadn't really changed much. I knew in my heart that I wouldn't want to continue with the pregnancy if there was any risk to my child, or me, but that would be the hardest decision I'd ever need to make. I'm not sure I could even contemplate another pregnancy if I were forced to terminate this pregnancy now. I didn't want to think about the scenarios but understood that this woman was only doing her job.

The test was a simple, straightforward blood test. The results were 99.5% accurate, but it would be the weeklong wait to hear either way that would be torment. I should be well and truly used to waiting by now, but each time I was faced with another timeframe it felt like another way of pounding on my anxieties. With this particular test, I had no prior experience. Every medical professional I had met so far has not helped with my heightened paranoia around the results. I am continually told that I'm a high-risk pregnancy with my age and my history. Over that week I continually played out what the conversation might sound like should the consultant call me with bad news. Yet, I really couldn't predict the results, and waiting was my only option. I kept telling myself that this pregnancy was the one; I kept pushing my mind to think positively. We had been through so much; surely this one thing would go our way? Although who was I to request special entitlement?

At almost eleven weeks I now felt pregnant. My body had started to change; albeit only slightly. My breasts were swollen and sore, and my belly was a little bloated, but certainly not showing a bump – yet. I couldn't wait until my stomach started growing, and becoming round. I started to anticipate that first moment when I'd feel my baby move inside of me. It was all a wonderful promise, and despite not wanting to build my hopes, I couldn't help but start to think ahead.

I was pleased that the test results came back at spot on five days. I had anxiously called the clinic the morning of the fifth day. I'm sure they get similar calls from other anxious women. I was told that it wasn't likely that the results would arrive that day, but she promised to phone me as soon as she received them. I graciously thanked her for her understanding and tried to concentrate on the rest of my day at work, but with little success.

It was only just before three o'clock in the afternoon when an unknown number came through on my mobile. I hadn't let go of my phone all day in the hope that the results would arrive earlier than expected. As I answered the call, my heart leapt when the same woman from earlier introduced herself. Thankfully, she quickly advised me that our results were good, that we had a healthy baby with no chromosomal abnormalities. My voice wavered as I thanked her profusely, feeling my eyes start to water with tears of relief. Another milestone passed! I could hardly believe our luck!

Then she asked me another question, "Would you like to know your baby's gender?"

Whilst my husband would have been happy to wait to find out, I was eager to know, and after much discussion we had agreed to find out the gender. In part, I wanted to share this information with my father, hoping it might give him the incentive to hold on to meet our new-born baby. In another sense, knowing the gender made the pregnancy more real for me, and it gave me hope that this time we would have our rainbow baby. Whatever the case, I quickly responded to her question with, 'Yes please!"

She laughed at my enthusiasm in a friendly manner. "You're having a boy," she said enthusiastically. "Congratulations, Rachel!"

"Thank you so much!" I replied, feeling myself choke with emotion.

This was good news; we had a healthy baby boy. Suddenly, it all started to feel real. As soon as I finished the call, I dialled my husband with our exciting news. We were both elated at the news that our baby was a little boy! This was a good day, and we were now just two weeks shy of reaching our second trimester. Whilst it still felt surreal, I had to let myself feel a little more confident, deciding that it was okay to be slightly excited at the prospect of being a mother at long last!

Weather Warning

We were leaving for Australia just after my thirteenth week of pregnancy, and I couldn't have been happier to return home with our good news. Despite the wretchedness of my father's condition, I had hope that this pregnancy would keep his spirits high and help him to focus positively over the coming months. He had now finished his radium treatment course, and in my last conversation with Mum she warned me that he was a little less himself. On the flight, I did wonder how different. With my dad it was hard at times, as he didn't talk much on the telephone anyway, so being in person and spending time with him would be the only way that I could truly understand how much the disease has really impacted on him.

It's a long flight to Australia and certainly not the most pleasant of journeys. Over twenty-four hours of travelling, stopovers and different time zones take their toll on any person. Being pregnant, it made the journey a little less comfortable, but I was glad that I was only still early on my pregnancy and so the discomfort was still at a minimum.

I had been lucky so far, with little nausea during my first trimester. The most I felt during that flight was a little tired and bloated. However, at the airport I noticed something else when I went to the bathroom. It was a strange feeling at first, as though I had left a tampon in (excuse the graphic visualisation), and of course I wasn't wearing anything down there, so I checked. At first, I really didn't know what I was dealing with, but there was definitely something strange going on. The best way I could describe it was a thick piece of skin inside my vagina. Again, it sounds so crude, but of course I worried. I went back to my husband who was enjoying a glass of champagne in the airport lounge. He too seemed completely baffled by what I described was protruding down there. With the flight being called in less than an hour, I wasn't sure what to do. Do we board, or was this something I should seek urgent medical attention for.

My first instinct was to seek out the response of a few of the trusted ladies I had connected with on a specific pregnancy social media group. Time was running out, and if we had to make a decision about this flight, we had to do it fast. I cursed my luck, as this was such bad timing. Postponing or cancelling flights wasn't something I could frivolously do, and whilst this was important, I also had to consider the cost both personally and financially if it turned out to be nothing at all. I kept telling myself that it wasn't painful and I wasn't bleeding, so it couldn't be an emergency. Nonetheless, my husband and I felt a little panicked to make a decision.

I know we shouldn't have, but we Googled, and I conversed on the forum, trying to explain the symptoms, seeking any type of explanation. The feedback I was getting was that this could be a cervical prolapse. I hadn't really heard of it, and surely it was too early in my pregnancy for such a thing? From what I could see, it seemed to be considered as a common occurrence in women who had undergone uterine surgeries in the past. None of them offered any solutions except to wait it out. Often the condition rectified itself. Everything I was finding told me that if there was no pain or bleeding that it was most likely not an emergency, but should be seen to if it didn't disappear.

We took the flight, knowing that we would be in Australia in around twenty-four hours, and I could monitor it along the journey. I still wasn't one hundred percent sure, but we had to make a decision, and my gut instinct told me that going to emergency wasn't going to solve the issue immediately. Had I not noticed it, physically, I wouldn't have even known it was there.

More than anything, I wanted to go home, see my dad and my family, and I could seek immediate medical attention when I arrived. This trip was too important on many levels, and whilst some may think me foolish, I had to go with my instincts. Arriving home into the warm Brisbane sun reassured me that I had made the right choice. My father was so excited to see us, and it was worth all that angst to finally be able to really hug him. He looked well. He was thinner, his hair had mostly fallen out, and he looked more fragile than I remembered, but he was my dad, and I was pleased we didn't cancel or postpone our flight.

Nothing had changed, for better or worse, with this condition that had formed, but I knew I had to get it seen to. However, I was somewhat relieved to have an uneventful flight, and whilst it hadn't gone away, I was able to now seek medical attention. Once I told my mother she jumped to action, arranging for an out of hours doctor to come to their home to see to my case. I was referred to the local hospital for further examination. It was all very easy and straightforward, and my Google investigative skills were correct; it was a prolapse of my cervix. There was nothing I could do about it, and as I suspected, with no bleeding or pain, they felt it was just something that may retract eventually, or as my pregnancy progressed would need further attention. They advised me that baby was probably pushing downwards, causing the prolapse, and that as he continued to grow and my uterus expand upwards, it was likely to release the pressure on my pelvic area. I was asked to monitor it, and to rest as much as possible.

If anything, it reassured me that we made the right decision by getting on that flight. I would have cursed myself had we lost the money and the opportunity to fly home, to hear that exact prognosis. So needless to say I was uncomfortable but at no risk. It was just another thing I had to face on this crazy journey but I kept telling myself that it would be all worth the anxiety in the end, when I finally meet my little man and get to hold him in my arms. These little tests along the way, whatever their purpose, just made me more determined to get to that end goal. It was hard to believe that we were finally in the second trimester, and one third of this pregnancy was complete. Still, it was a long road ahead, and I had to stay patient and positive.

Whilst I couldn't partake in many of the activities we would normally plan for a summer holiday in Australia, we enjoyed a relaxing break with my family with trips to the beach, enjoying the warm sunshine. It was the end of summer, but it was still incredibly warm. My husband, who is from Northern Ireland, found the weather particularly toasty. I was starting to form a small bump. Most people would probably think I had an extra large lunch, but I knew it was my little man growing inside me. I was able to mostly wear my normal clothes, but with my tummy slightly expanding, my shorts and trousers needed to have some give. It was exciting to start to see my body changing before me, and in those few weeks that we were in Australia, it definitely felt as though I had a small growth spurt.

Every day, I checked my own condition too. Whilst the doctors had assured me that there was no immediate risk with my cervix having prolapsed, I wanted to ensure that it didn't get worse. Nothing changed for almost two weeks, and it became a habit each morning and night for me to check. Without warning, however, just over fourteen days since I first noticed the prolapse, and coming up to week fifteen of the pregnancy, it was gone. It hadn't just moved; it had completely disappeared. It was so strange, and I certainly wasn't complaining, but I was relieved. I could genuinely relax into the last week of our vacation in Australia, knowing that whatever it was, things were still progressing nicely in our pregnancy.

I wanted to do something for my dad whilst we were in town, something to get him excited about my pregnancy, to help him focus on staying strong, and perhaps give him the willpower to keep fighting until his newest grandson arrived. So my Mum and I booked a private scan. The clinic we found was designed especially for relatives and families who wanted to view a new pregnancy, and so it was perfect. It was just my husband, my mum and dad, and myself. The set up was fantastic, arranged like a mini movie theatre, with our little baby in the lead role. The ultrasound scans were something that my parents never had when they were expecting, so this was also a new experience for them.

It was truly amazing! My little man was wiggling about; he gave them a high five, and we could see all of his little fingers, and I almost wept as both my parents were completely overwhelmed by the physical details they could see on the screen in front of them. At only just past fifteen weeks, he was almost perfectly formed, and the sonographer took her time, ensuring that they were able to get a good picture of their grandson-to-be. We had a video made, and I gifted that to my parents as a keepsake. I was so pleased to have been able to share that moment with them, and I know it meant a lot to my father, who couldn't stop talking about it for days after. It was a perfect moment for all of us.

Torrential Downpour

Saying good-bye to my dad was more than difficult. We had thoroughly enjoyed our time back home, and it was wonderful to see my family, spending quality time with my dad. I was now just shy of sixteen weeks, and my parents were able to see the small growing bump, and of course the scan. After everything we had been through to get to this pregnancy, they too were hopeful that this was finally our time to be parents. For my dad, I hoped that this would be enough to give him the willpower to make it until he could meet his little grandson. I knew I couldn't keep him alive forever, and that this cancer was limiting his time, but I truly hoped I could get one more chance to see him in person again. Next time I hoped to hand him a little grandson to hold. It is those moments that are so incredibly precious, and I only needed one more. I prayed on the plane to Sydney that this one wish would be granted.

This pregnancy was truly a blessing, but in terms of timing, it would now be challenging for me to travel again back to Australia before my baby was born. Skype and phone calls would have to suffice, but they weren't quite the same as a real human hug.

My husband and I stopped through in Sydney for two nights before our departure to London. He had never been to the state capital before, and given our flight connections, it was a good excuse to do a little sightseeing. I left Brisbane with a heavy heart, promising my dad that I would return shortly after the birth so he could hold his grandson. I hoped I could fulfil that promise.

Arriving in Sydney, the weather was incredibly warm. We checked into our lovely boutique hotel, right by Sydney Harbour, and quickly set out to walk and explore. I hadn't been in the city for years, so it was fun to wander around and reacquaint myself with the sights. We had a big lunch, and it was a long day of walking. As the evening approached, my legs were tired, and we both felt hot and bothered from the heat. We decided on an early dinner at the hotel bar. Just some small starters in a more relaxed setting suited us both perfectly, as we would be up early the next morning for more sightseeing.

As we sat there conversing, I said to my husband, "I know I've been paranoid up to this point, and I'm sorry."

He leaned across and held my hand. "It's all good, though," he said reassuringly. "I'm positive."

I nodded, "Me too!" I really did feel that way, I thought to myself.

For the first time, I felt a little more relaxed about this pregnancy, and a new confidence was building as it dawned on me. *This could actually happen!* I smiled and sat back in the lounge in the small bar in the hotel, contentedly sipping my hot chocolate, whilst my husband enjoyed his beer.

We sat there talking for a while longer before deciding it was best to get an early night. Oh how times had changed, and certainly pregnancy itself didn't help. We laughed at ourselves as we checked the time. It was just after nine-thirty. It didn't matter, though; we were quite happy to shower and find a movie to watch in our hotel room before a full night's rest.

My husband went to the bathroom first, as I started fishing through my suitcase for my pyjamas. Suddenly I froze on the spot, sucked my breath in as I felt something. Without thinking, I shoved my hand down my trousers and into my underwear. I was wet! When I brought my hand out I wailed in dismay. It was blood, and a lot of it.

"What? What's happened?" My husband called in panic from behind the closed bathroom door.

I couldn't say anything. I just cried, staring at my hand, feeling more wetness between my legs. The bathroom door opened, and I raced inside, past my husband who was confused by my distress and panic. I was definitely bleeding, and there was a lot of it.

"I'm bleeding!" I cried out. "It's heavy!"

"What?"

"I just felt it, it just started," I sobbed, as I watched it fill up the toilet bowl. My hopes began to crash as I suddenly felt all of that confidence and hope I had just talked about begin to disappear.

My husband stood in the doorway helpless to the situation. I looked up at him and broke down into tears. "We need to get to a hospital..." I said feebly.

He nodded; his eyes said it all. There was too much blood. There was more than I had ever experienced in my early miscarriages. We both felt it was over, or it was going. Just like that, with no warning at all.

I had nothing with me, so I had to use toilet paper as I dressed to leave the hotel. My husband called a taxi, and the hotel receptionist gave us the details for the nearest hospital emergency. I couldn't talk. I couldn't even look my husband in the eyes. He held my hand in the back of the cab the entire way as I sobbed.

The nurse who took our details was kind. She went to get me some sanitary towels and told us a doctor would see us as soon as possible. We didn't have to wait long before we were taken into another waiting room. My blood pressure was taken, and I had finally calmed down enough to explain my history. There were a lot of others also in the emergency department that night, so we were asked to take a seat in a room alongside many others of all ages, with all different sorts of ailments.

We had to wait our turn. I found myself going to the bathroom regularly to check. The bleeding was starting to slow down, which was good, but it still didn't comfort me. We sat and waited for a couple of hours. I didn't expect them to rush us through; there were much more serious cases ahead of me. However, as I sat there I contemplated how I would manage another loss. This would be so much harder than the other four miscarriages. My body had started to change, and, at just under sixteen weeks I was far more attached to this pregnancy; the little baby boy who was now a fully formed foetus inside my belly. I sat there and wept as we waited. My husband was quiet too. He held my hand, stroked my arm, and gave me a gentle kiss on the cheek every now and then. We were both anxious and scared. This was the last place we had expected to be, and yet as time passed, I started to reconcile to myself that I would be returning to the UK without the promise of a baby in our future. Just thinking about it sent me into a fit of sobs. I wasn't sure how I could recover from this. We had come too far this time. It was so much harder to contemplate that we might lose this baby too!

Finally, we were called to see a doctor. I was brought into a very small examination room. The bleeding had now subsided, but I went through my full history with her, including the recent prolapsed cervix just over two weeks earlier. She wasn't a gynaecologist but she performed an internal examination. There was little she could see, and couldn't confirm either way what was happening. I was told to wait again in the main room, whilst she sought some further advice. Another hour passed before we were called back again. It was past midnight now, and I was tired, emotional and exhausted.

"It's good news that your bleeding has stopped," the doctor suggested.

I refused to give myself any false hope, but I nodded and tried to smile. We were told that a scan would confirm for sure if the bleed meant that the pregnancy was ending. She did say that the bleeding could be a result of my cervical prolapse. I wasn't convinced; surely the bleeding would have happened at the time or immediately after. The pregnancy unit was closed and we were told to come back in the morning first thing, to get a scan. I was offered a hospital bed for the night, but declined. I wanted to go back to the hotel and sleep, hold my husband. I didn't care that we would be returning in just a few hours; right at that moment I needed space. The doctor understood and asked us to wait until she wrote up her report.

As we waited inside the small consulting room, I apologised to my husband. "I'm sorry!"

"What are you sorry for?" he asked me in surprise.

"This is your first time in Sydney and I've ruined it." I knew in my heart what I was saying made no sense, but my heart was heavy with sorrow, and despite everything we had been through I had really started to think positively about this pregnancy.

"Don't say that," he chastised. "None of this is your fault, and we don't know for sure that you are losing this baby. You heard the doctor. We have to wait for the scan." He was always the ever-hopeful one, and I nodded but I didn't feel that hope. He knew I didn't believe him. "We will come back first thing in the morning, yes?" he said softly, moving his head so that he could meet my eyes. I nodded again. The department would open in a few hours. I doubted I would sleep before then, but it would at least prepare me to hear the words that I had heard before. I needed to prepare myself for the fall.

The doctor came back into the room after a while. "Do you mind waiting just a little bit longer? I have spoken about your case to one of our gynaecologists, and she wants to see what we can do tonight."

We both nodded. Neither of us were sure what could be done at this hour of the night, but we were here now, and I was open to anything.

Another thirty minutes passed before another woman knocked on the door. She introduced herself, a specialist in gynaecology, and asked if she could examine me. She told us the same thing as the doctor; only a scan could confirm for sure what was happening. I wasn't surprised, but thanked her. She asked us to wait, that she would be back with us shortly. Again I was confused. What were we waiting for now? I was too tired to become impatient, but I started to feel that the night was dragging out. We didn't have to wait long again before she re-entered the small room. Behind her was another woman, a nurse, with a large mobile machine.

"I'm not sure why this wasn't offered to you earlier, but we can do a scan now," the gynaecologist proclaimed.

"Really? Thank you!" I burbled.

Whilst I knew this could be the confirmation of the end of this pregnancy, at least I could start grieving properly. The machine was wheeled into the room. There was barely enough room for it with me in the examination bed, my husband and the doctor. They manoeuvred things about to get it into position.

"You are almost sixteen weeks?" The gynaecologist asked. I nodded. "Okay, we should definitely be able to tell what is happening," she said reassuringly, as she lifted my top and started up the machine. I closed my eyes and held my breath as the device moved over my belly. My husband squeezed my hand. "Well we have a strong beating heart!" she told us both straight away and my eyes sprang open to look at the small black and white monitor.

"Really? He is ok?" I gasped.

"Yes, your baby is looking good," she said, smiling.

"But the bleeding?" I questioned.

"Your placenta is quite low, and given you had a cervical prolapse, it could be a blood clot caused by that. It's a condition that many women have in their pregnancies and it can cause bleeding," she explained. "I've examined you, and your cervix is closed, and there are no signs of bleeding inside the uterus which are all good signs."

My heart raced, and I felt a massive wave of relief sweep over me. I wanted to cry again, but this time it would be tears of joy. I was still pregnant. He was okay. It just didn't seem real!

The gynaecologist touched my shoulder, "I'm glad we could put you at ease tonight." I was so grateful to her I couldn't express it, I just smiled, and my husband thanked her. "You are flying back to the UK when?" she asked us.

"On Sunday," my husband answered, it was less than two days.

She looked a little concerned. "Okay, take it easy, nothing strenuous over the next two days, and if you have any further bleeding you come straight back to the hospital," she warned us. "On the flight, try to stay comfortable, and again, no lifting heavy suitcases, and I suggest you go to a specialist on your return to the UK."

We both nodded, still smiling stupidly. I wasn't going to do anything to risk this, so I took her advice under strict instruction.

Sunshine on a Rainy Day

My husband became my personal gatekeeper for the rest of our time in Sydney. We did take it easy, and despite my protests that he could do some sightseeing alone, he was also determined to remain by my side. I was grateful, as I felt drained, emotionally and physically, from our night in the emergency ward. We booked a boat tour around Sydney's harbour, which involved not much but sitting in the sunshine and taking lots of photos. We didn't go far from the hotel otherwise, but luckily we were staying in a central location.

There was no more bleeding, but the paranoia and anxiety had returned. This pregnancy was not without its drama, and I had to accept that it might never be a straightforward, easy journey. We had passed yet another hurdle, and my emotions were still raw. Just shy of sixteen weeks, we were closer to reaching the half way point, but there was still a long way to go, and with each day I felt more invested in the little man growing inside me. The scare we had told me that it would be even harder now should things go wrong.

The flight home was uneventful and long, and I was prepared to return to work just a day after landing. I followed the instructions of the gynaecologist and booked in to see my specialist within days of returning. He confirmed what she had suspected. I had a low-lying placenta, which therefore could result in further bleeding. It was also likely I would need to be monitored under consultant care throughout the remainder of my pregnancy. However, I was able to see our baby once again, as he scanned me and I was given further reassurance as I watched my little boy wiggle and move about and heard his strong beating heart. Everything was looking perfect.

I did have another small bleed that week, but this time I didn't panic. Like before, it stopped within a few hours, and I didn't even go to hospital. I wasn't sure how I would cope if it occurred regularly, but I was satisfied for the time being that everything was generally okay with my baby and that it was a similar occurrence to the episode in Sydney.

Even though I was reassured, I still felt that there was a dark cloud hanging over my head with this pregnancy. As I told a few friends what happened, I could almost feel them sigh in frustration for me. I felt like a pregnant basket case, a drama queen. I wanted desperately to enjoy being pregnant and the miracle that was growing inside me. However, I just couldn't. I had tried relaxing that night in the hotel bar with my husband, and yet less than an hour later after I had proclaimed my confidence, I was heading to emergency. It sometimes felt as though I was being told I couldn't get comfortable, that I had to stay on guard the entire time.

I had my first midwife appointment in the weeks that followed. I was seventeen weeks at that stage. She was surprised I had left it so late to have my first appointment, and also asked me why I had private scans up until this point. I felt a little silly explaining my paranoia, but she was truly wonderful. For the first time in the public system in the United Kingdom, I felt supported. It was a vast difference from the very first midwife I had met in my first pregnancy. I was pleased to have changed the doctor's surgery, and I was grateful for her understanding and support. We spoke about booking myself into hospitals, and again, given my past experiences I felt a little unsure about returning to the local hospital. It sounds crazy, but in some ways I felt that I had only experienced loss and further complications from my experiences locally, and I was hesitant to tempt fate. Again she reassured me that my anxieties were real, and suggested another hospital that was also close by, just another five minutes away. Her encouragement filled me with hope, and I was comforted by her reassurance that my case was higher risk and therefore I could expect more monitoring and care throughout.

Within days, I had a letter from the hospital we had chosen inviting me to attend an appointment with a specialist consultant. Perhaps my expectations were low from past experience, but I was pleasantly surprised by my experience within this new hospital from day one. It was also part of the National Health Service, but the difference in care, attention and general experience was miles apart from the hospital I had been using previously. Of course, there were still wait times, but they weren't excessive, and the nurses, reception staff and my consultant were all helpful, supportive and empathetic to my history. I was put on a regular schedule of scans to monitor growth throughout my pregnancy, and the consultant understood my history, explaining some of the risks I may face throughout the pregnancy, but reassuring me that she would do her best to ensure the safe arrival of our baby boy. I couldn't have asked for more. Despite everything I had experienced, I felt that I was getting the best possible care moving forward. Everything else was really down to fate.

Given my age, the complications and potential risks, I was advised that I should expect to be booked in for a caesarean section at around thirty-eight or thirty-nine weeks. I know many women have an ideal surrounding the birth of their child and what that experience should look like. For me, I just wanted to hold my little boy and know he was safe and sound. I told my consultant that I would take her advice, and I wouldn't question it. It was all about what was right for the baby and me. I liked her. She was honest and encouraging, and she made me feel safe. I felt my trust and faith in the public system quickly being restored with those few interactions, and I knew I would be a regular visitor at this hospital with appointments and scans scheduled every two weeks. At least I could watch our little man grow with the knowledge that if anything were to happen, it would be caught quickly.

Staying Indoors

One thing I have noticed since being pregnant is that suddenly my social life has become somewhat absent. It's certainly not from lack of trying on my part, but it is obvious that friends now make a general assumption that I won't be interested in parties or events. Last year, I had regular invites to dinners out, parties, events; this year, barely anything.

I'm not complaining, it's merely an observation. I was scanning a baby forum for my birth month the other day, and this exact topic came up. It seems I'm not alone. Perhaps people assume that I cannot be around alcohol, loud noise or even enjoy a late night out. Of course, I'm not looking to rave into the early hours of the morning, but I certainly miss the standard socialising with my friends and colleagues. I'm not afraid of being in a pub and drinking soda water; heaven forbid I'm around someone who may be a little intoxicated.

Whilst my body is changing, and I am now starting to feel a lot more tired as I get closer to my third trimester, I have wanted this social interaction. Yet, how do you approach this subject? I was talking to my husband, who is generally quite upfront and straightforward, about my concerns. He told me to just speak to my friends. Sounded easy enough, but I certainly didn't want to accuse them of isolating me. To be honest, I'm not sure they are even doing it consciously. Perhaps I've even done the same to my pregnant friends in the past?

I know that there are different expectations of me now as I prepare for motherhood. I certainly wouldn't trade my position for anything, and it's not as though I begrudge anyone for how I'm feeling, but at times it is lonely. I have plenty of friends with children who are welcoming me to brunches or lunches, and giving me advice and tips on parenting, preparing me for this huge life change. However, I watch the social media posts of dinner parties, weekends away and night's out, and I wonder if I'm ever a thought when the invites are extended. How do you ask that question? Even more so, will I be back on that invite list again one day?

It's certainly not the biggest issue I've had to face during this pregnancy, but it's something that has started to play on my mind over the past few months. Most people would tell me that motherhood changes your perspective on your social life, and I understand that and I am willing to embrace being a mother with open arms. However, I'm never going to be the woman who cannot leave her child. There will be times where I will need a small break, time away, whether it is shopping, catching up with friends or a night out. In my own personal view, I want to ensure that my husband has his moments alone to bond with our baby, giving me the opportunity to meet with friends or just take a personal moment. It irks me when people say their husband is babysitting, like it's not his job to be a parent? Of course I understand that my socialising will be incredibly diminished compared to what it has been in the past. That's a given. However, for me, it's about balance. I will be a better mother because I am who I am. I need to strike a healthy balance, and find a pattern that works.

What I do find surprising is that it seems to be a given that I'm written out of these social events already. I guess there is an assumption that I won't want to leave the house for the first six months, and it sometimes feels as though this decision to opt in or out of events has been taken away from me. It's not everyone, and it's not just friends. Colleagues and acquaintances even comment on any plans I discuss post birth, sometimes scoffing that I will change my mind when this baby arrives. Perhaps it's just my paranoia, and I realise that I can't partake in some of these events, but I want to make that choice. At the moment, it's mainly teas, brunches or lunches, which of course I enjoy, but as far as parties and other more exciting events, it feels as though I'm no longer considered a participant.

Even when I have mentioned a night out, I sometimes feel that eyebrows are raised cynically, and I've not pushed this. *Should I really be taking it this personally?* To be truthful, I'm not sure how I really feel. I certainly hope it's just a pregnancy phase; that when baby arrives, these trivial concerns will no longer matter. Time will tell.

The Sound of Thunder

Having experienced loss previously and with all the challenges we have faced, it was hard to appease the anxiety throughout this pregnancy. So many people have told me that I should relax and stay positive – that's easier said than done. I continued to remind myself that we had passed our biggest milestones, and yet as I looked ahead there was still a distance to travel, and I had heard and read so many horror stories of late losses, emergency pre-term labour and more. Forty weeks is a very long time, especially when you are growing a little human and literally counting each day until you can hold them.

We had finally reached the halfway point of this pregnancy. A major milestone, but yet I kept thinking that I needed to stay positive for another twenty weeks! If only time could just move a little faster?

At this stage of the pregnancy, we had our anomaly scan booked. It was a thorough investigation of all the baby's organs, bone structure, growth and an opportunity to pre-empt any issues. We had been having scans fortnightly up to this point, so I wasn't worried about growth. In fact, he was always measuring slightly ahead, which reassured me that our baby was healthy, but would be big and tall by the time he arrived. My husband is tall, and so am I, so that was to be expected. In a way, I felt comfortable with the caesarean section being booked, as my nephews were born around nine pounds each. I almost shuddered each time I thought of how I could push that out naturally – but people do!

We had the Harmony blood screening for abnormalities at ten weeks, so going into this scan I hadn't expected any hiccups. Finally, I was feeling much more at ease entering those small ultrasound rooms, and the hospital we had booked into had a myriad of staff that would always openly explain their findings during each procedure. It made the world of difference as an anxious, expectant mum, and even their general conversation and welcome each time reinforced that we had made the right choice to switch.

My husband came with me for the scan. It had been difficult for him to take time off for each appointment prior to this. I was a frequent visitor to the hospital with my scan, consultant and antenatal appointments, but this ultrasound was different.

Everything seemed to be looking positive. His growth was on track, slightly ahead but not concerning. No structural concerns with his spine, neck, head, and good blood flow through the heart, brain and other organs. His bladder was fine, and facial features showed no signs of anything other than normal. His arms, fingers and thighbones were structurally normal and all a good length. He was moving quite a bit, and it took a while, but when the sonographer stopped at his feet we knew there was something amiss.

Straight away she stopped, took a few still images and moved in closer to examine. "It appears as though your baby may have bilateral Talipes," she explained as she peered closer to the screen, zooming the image in. The small room had a monitor on display so that I could watch what she was doing, and I couldn't make out much of what was showing in the black and white pictures. I looked at my husband and he shrugged his shoulders.

"What's that?" I asked softly, a little confused.

"It's the medical term for club feet," she answered. "Do you mind waiting here a minute? I just need to get someone in to have a look, for a second opinion, if that's ok?"

I could only nod in agreement as I lay there, not really sure what to say; I hadn't heard much about club feet before or what it meant. I looked at my husband and he held my hand. After she had left the room, we waited just a few minutes before another sonographer returned with our lady. The new sonographer sat in front of the screen, and started wiggling the scanning device around on my tummy.

"Yes, it's definitely Talipes," the lady said. "I can see the condition on both feet."

I could only nod. I was in shock, but also completely confused. I had no idea if this was good, bad or in the middle. I could see my husband on his phone. He was clearly googling the term to get more information. The new sonographer continued to look at my baby's legs, spine and did a re-scan on what the first sonographer had covered.

They came back to the brain. "Ok, so all the brain chambers look good, and there are no immediate concerns. However, I can see a small choroid plexus cyst." I felt my heart stop as the sonographer spoke, and my anxiety building even further. "Look," she said quickly, as she must have seen the panic in my eyes, "we don't normally note these on our scans. Many babies actually have them; in fact, the statistics are around one in a hundred. They are small and often they disappear. However, given the Talipes diagnosis, I'm obliged to mention any other markers." Her justification didn't make me feel any calmer.

As she spoke, my mind whirred with questions, but I just couldn't speak. Club feet, sounded bad. I had to admit that it was something I had very limited knowledge of, and didn't fully understand. However, a cyst on his brain? I felt completely overwhelmed. The sonographer was kind and sympathetic, and explained that we would be booked to see a foetal medical specialist to get more information.

When she finally left the small scan room, I looked at my husband.

"Let's just see what they tell us." He was pre-empting my panic, and remaining calm. That's what he does. He always seems to be the sensible one in these situations.

Once I had dressed, we were taken to a small room where a nurse greeted us. As we sat down she handed us a handful of printouts and a small card. "I'm sorry you've had this diagnosis," she said sincerely, "but the information I've handed you will give you much more information about Talipes, and this card, it's a counselling service. They can give you some guidance and advice, perhaps even some reassurance." I nodded gratefully. "I'm booking you in for a follow up appointment with a specialist, who will recheck the results, but will also talk to you about what happens next."

"What causes this?" I asked.

Shaking her head, she said, "It could be genetics, positioning or there could be something else. You will be offered an amniocentesis test to check for any other disabilities," she added.

"We had the Harmony test," I said quickly. "It showed low risk."

"Yes, and whether you decide to have the amniocentesis test is completely your choice. It may give you additional information or reassurance."

I didn't understand. Surely the test we did at ten weeks was sufficient? I had paid over five hundred pounds for this test so that I didn't have to have the amniocentesis test. One was supposed to negate the other. I had heard so many negative reports about the amniocentesis, and I didn't want this test. It had a risk of miscarriage, and I had to wonder what it would tell me that the Harmony test didn't. I needed to further understand and balance out the risks. I couldn't make this decision right now. I needed time.

"And this cyst?" I asked tentatively.

"It may be nothing. We rarely even report on those markers anymore. However, your baby has Talipes, and so it is something we do need to mention. It's what we call a soft marker. It may be a sign that your baby has a trisomy or another disability, something that may be detected at birth. The amniocentesis may be able to detect this pre-birth. Or the two markers may be completely separate."

I still didn't understand fully. "And the feet? What can they do?"

"We have some very good specialists here in the hospital. Depending on the severity, we would suggest a treatment plan as soon as he is born, which would include physiotherapy, casting of the foot into position and potentially braces. All this can be done whilst he is very young and whilst his bones are still soft. It's a very treatable condition."

She was helpful, and her words started to calm me, but I still had hundreds of questions. I just couldn't pull them out of my head now. I needed time to digest these results. I wanted time alone with my husband to talk to him. We were given a follow up appointment for the next week.

Of course, as soon as we left the hospital my husband and I googled Talipes and Choroid Plexus Cysts. Wrong move! Some of the stories were concerning. With the feet, we found a lot of wonderful stories of rehabilitation, even sports stars who've been born with the condition, but early treatment meant that it never impacted their physical ability to walk, run and compete. That was reassuring at least. It was this second soft marker – the choroid plexus cyst – throwing a curve ball into the equation. On its own, it was a minuscule issue, most of which said it disappeared or meant nothing. In fact, many adults develop these and never know otherwise. However, it was the two 'soft markers' together as they termed this; the Talipes and the cyst, which sent my anxieties skyward. Many stories said it went away, meant nothing. Other stories were more concerning, telling of birth defects, disabilities, and abnormalities. I had thought we had crossed off these risks with the early Harmony test but now I suddenly doubted everything I knew. I touched my growing belly as I felt him wiggle inside me, and I could only pray that it was just the feet.

I called the counselling number that afternoon. Sitting down on my bed, I explained what we had been told, what the scan had revealed and the information we had been given. The woman on the phone listened kindly; I knew that she probably had dozens of calls like this every day. I told her of the option given to us to undergo a further testing with the amniocentesis test. However, I had already researched this and there was a one to two percent risk of miscarrying with this test. Of course, I was nervous about even considering this, given my history. At only twenty weeks pregnant, my baby couldn't survive if he was suddenly forced into an early labour. Weighing up the pros and cons of undergoing this test was a difficult decision, and my husband and I had no idea which was the less risky option.

I knew the woman on the phone couldn't tell me what to do, but just having someone to talk through everything seemed to offload the anxiety that was quickly building inside of me.

"What would you do if the amnio test came back with a disability?" she asked me.

I paused a second. I had to contemplate that this could be a reality. "I'm not sure. I would want to know if there was anything wrong that was life threatening to my baby..." I let my thoughts spill out.

"From what you have told me, there are no other indicators of anything serious with your baby," she said. "You told me his heart, back, lungs, legs all came back with no issues?"

"Yes," I said hopefully.

"So, if you were to do the amnio test, I would assume by what you said, that if there was a disability, it wouldn't be life threatening?" she put to me, in a way that almost answered my own question. "At twenty weeks, severe abnormalities can often be detected in the scan and your Harmony test also came back with low risk results," she added reassuringly.

As I contemplated her words, I could feel my heartbeat slowing to a normal pace, and the scenario seemed to make much more sense. "So if I were to have the test, it may show something, but it's most likely something that a child could live with?" I questioned, but I was primarily talking to myself out loud.

"That is the possibility. Or there is nothing else at all, and your baby just has Talipes ..." she said softly. "The decision you would be asked if there was something, is whether it is something you would want to terminate this pregnancy over."

I shook my head vigorously. I knew she couldn't see me, but in my mind, I couldn't go back now, not even if my baby did have a small disability. Especially if it wasn't life threatening. "No, I couldn't." I knew that for certain. I couldn't let go of my baby now. He was mine. I could feel him move inside me as we spoke, and there was no debate in my mind.

"I think you are coming to your own decision," the woman spoke softly. "You need to weigh up the risk of this amnio test and what may happen should it spark an early labour. At twenty weeks, your baby won't survive that. If you did do the test, and you found out something more about your baby, the next question would be whether you would you continue with your pregnancy."

It sounded so simple, and in a way it was. The test itself was just going to prepare me more than anything; it wasn't going to solve anything. I touched my belly again. I had wished for this baby for so long, and for twenty weeks now he has been growing inside me. I loved him already. I couldn't risk losing him. He was mine, for better or for worse. We would travel this road together and I would face the odds when the time comes.

"Thank you," I said to the woman. "You've helped me process this. I think I don't want to do any further testing... I mean, I'm not sure how it would change the future of this pregnancy? But, I know I wouldn't do anything now at this stage... Unless of course it was life threatening. But if anything were life threatening, they would have found something to indicate that, right?" I was thinking out loud again as I spoke to her, but as before, it helped me to manage my thoughts.

"Yes, I'd say so," the woman confirmed. "I'm glad I helped, and I truly wish you the best with this pregnancy," she concluded positively.

Immediately after I hung up the phone I called my husband and replayed the conversation. He and I both agreed, we couldn't take the risk on this test. We had come this far, and we had to let fate play its hand. At this stage, we could only hope that it was only our baby's little feet. If the prognosis turned out to be more than just his feet, that there were further health or physical concerns, we would cross that bridge when our son was born. The storm wasn't over, but it was starting to become easier to weather.

Finding a Path Through the Fog

I had to wonder how I would get through the next twenty weeks of this pregnancy, and how many more knockbacks I could handle. Pregnancy is supposed to be a wonderful time for an expectant mother, a time to enjoy every change in your body as you prepare for that life-changing experience. I couldn't help but want to fast forward it all. I wanted to enjoy it but I just couldn't. I wanted to get to the end and hold my baby. All these obstacles just kept knocking my confidence. I wanted to know that my baby would be alright.

My husband and I talked over the diagnosis of our son's feet, as well as this vague choroid plexus cyst. After much advice and guidance, we felt a little less anxious about the cyst. Anything in the brain was always worrying, and so naturally I had to wonder whether it would impact my son's development or mental abilities. Apparently, however, it is extremely common. Many adults have them completely undetected, with no impact on brain functionality, development or other problems. In most cases the cyst disappears before birth. The only consideration that kept nagging at me was that the diagnosis considers this as two markers, and with that, does it increase the odds of there being a significant problem?

However, we had had the Harmony test, and the anomaly scan showed no signs of any other deformities; so we had to feel confident that there was nothing 'life-threatening', nothing we couldn't handle once our little boy was born. We had to be strong, and focus on the positive. We had made it to twenty weeks – half way – and we were literally on the home stretch. Therefore, whatever we found out now would make no difference to my decision to continue the pregnancy. We would manage, and most of all, we would love our son with every inch of our hearts, supporting him through whatever he needed, knowing that we were blessed to be granted a child, despite all of our challenges. At the end of the day, we would be parents, and our son would love us and we would love him, unconditionally. This was our dream.

I joined a Talipes group on social media and found an incredible community of support from other women who had also dealt with the condition with their children, as well as others who were currently going through corrective treatment. They shared photos and wrote about their experiences, which comforted me. I was able to look at babies born with clubfeet, those undergoing treatment, as well as children who many years after treatment were going on to win athletics awards and live perfectly normal lives.

Every now and then I would regress following that scan. I'd have moments, where I would panic about what could be, and I'd worry for the baby growing in my belly. My husband would catch me on the Internet and threaten to confiscate the computer, but for me it was the waiting, the not knowing and the guessing that started to take over my sanity. Having the Talipes group on social media would sometimes help. Many other women like me had also just received a similar diagnosis and were at a similar stage of their pregnancy. Hearing that I wasn't the only one panicking made me feel a little more comforted; that my emotions were actually natural. However, I did realise that I had to find a way to control my panic and anxiety, as I still had another half of this pregnancy to go. For the sake of my baby boy, I had to find a way to reconcile our decision against the amniocentesis test, knowing that I was leaving any further diagnosis up to fate. I had to be prepared for whatever may come when our little man was born, and accept that. To be very frank, once I made that decision, I felt a relief wash over me. There was no question of whether I would love and cherish my beautiful baby once he was born, regardless of any diagnosis. He was mine now. I'd carried and nurtured him for twenty weeks and

I'd nurture him for the rest of his life if I had to. I was a mum in every sense now; there was no going back.

Dressing for the Weather

I had often heard stories from other women about the perceptions they'd faced during their pregnancies. I guess I'd always shrugged them off as just that, perceptions. Many women had told me, warned me even, that priorities change once you're pregnant, and your prospects start to change too when it comes to career and work. Naively, I always assumed that I would be different.

Becoming a mother has been the ultimate dream of mine for years now, and I had also assumed that I could easily balance this with my career and ambitions. When we discovered that we were pregnant again just before Christmas, it was my ultimate dream come true. Once I'd settled into this pregnancy, and felt a level of comfort that it was progressing positively, I started to let myself make plans around maternity leave, career and a future with my baby. A strong part of me wanted to spend quality time with our baby, and we had enough savings for the time that I would have off work unpaid. I didn't want to feel that I had to rush back to work, although I wasn't quite sure if I would take the full twelve months leave I was entitled to. Already, I started to explore childcare options, as I knew eventually I would want to return to work. I knew I would want to ensure I could balance my family and my career effectively.

I had never proclaimed that I would be a full-time mum, and I knew in my heart that I would not be me if I compromised on that. Therefore, it was never a consideration that I would give up work completely. Although I also appreciate that this a choice factor for women. There is no absolute right or wrong here, and there also should never be any judgment. My mum was a working mum and I was never neglected, and so I knew I had it in me to maintain the balance I needed to prioritise both parts of my life – career and family.

However, what has been a real surprise for me in this pregnancy are the reactions and assumptions made before I've even left work. I guess many generalise based on their own experiences, their families and lifestyles. However, at this stage, I really didn't know how I would react to becoming a mother and taking that long sabbatical from work. Generally, I'm not known for slowing down. This would be a major life change for me – in a good way of course – but it would take some adapting to.

Having grown up with a working career mother was inspiring to me. My mum always had projects and different jobs going from as early as I can remember. My parents owned a bakery when I was very young. Some of my earliest memories are built from behind the counter watching my mother decorate cakes, serving customers or doing the finances for that small beachside bakery. Sometimes I thought I was helping; mostly I was getting in her way! Aside from that, my mother was a qualified high school teacher and also did some part-time work selling educational books to schools and nurseries. She balanced three children with a career, sometimes study and anything else she could fill her time with, whilst also maintaining the household. I can't remember her ever really stopping, and perhaps that's where I get my restless ambition? One thing I do know is that she always made time to help with my homework, proofread my assignments and read me a bedtime story. That's the mum I want to be.

I'm not sure how exactly I will react when my son arrives, but I do intend to return to work at some stage. On top of that, I also intend to keep writing and publishing books. The world of writing has become somewhat of a release for me, and I love the new connections I've made across the author community. I may not be able to operate at the pace I do today, but I am still determined to maintain these ambitions, if anything, to give my son a strong female role model. More than that, it is about being real to myself. I can't be someone I'm not, and for me, the best mother I can be – is to be me!

What I've found quite strange is how people start to talk to you differently once you start growing a small human. Regardless of how I want to be perceived, suddenly the conversation switches from business and work priorities, to nappies, sleep patterns and coping mechanisms. Everyone loves to share personal parenting stories (and nightmares), and I found myself desperately trying to divert the conversation back to normality. Whilst I was preparing myself for parenthood, I sometimes preferred to avoid the stories, as each baby is different, and we would cope in our own way. More than anything, I wanted to separate this from my work and my corporate life. I knew that me as a career person and me as a mother me were two different people. I felt that I was being given space and excuses were being made on my behalf. Some were even deciding for me that I would be tired, less motivated and less driven when I returned to work. It became frustrating, as suddenly I felt like a puppet on a string, and my choices were not being taken seriously.

Whilst opportunities were still given to me to take on projects and tasks, I found that many would almost assume that I would be slower, less driven and perhaps less interested in such tasks as my pregnancy progressed. I even had times where I was left off meetings, as people assumed I would be checking out, or not interested as the discussions were focused on future work deliverables. Balancing career and family was something I assumed was a personal choice, yet it felt that the choice was no longer mine. It felt as though there were people around deciding for me, advising me to just sit back and relax through the next few months before my maternity leave. It was an incredibly strange experience.

Don't get me wrong, I was appreciative of the thought, and in some ways it did give me the flexibility I needed to attend the ridiculous number of medical appointments being scheduled for me throughout this pregnancy. Yet still I found myself seeking out projects and work, and vying to get involved in challenging assignments in and out of work. Perhaps it was my way of trying to forget about the time that seemed to be lagging as I progressed through the pregnancy. Another thought was that it was my way of telling myself that life was still normal, that I was able to carry on like I could before. If anything, being busy kept my mind occupied and away from the anxieties of this pregnancy. Work was good therapy for me.

Dancing in the Rain

Throughout this entire pregnancy I have felt so overly cautious and sometimes unnecessarily anxious about what 'could' happen. Perhaps I sound pessimistic, but deep down, I have found it so hard to believe that I could actually, finally get my rainbow baby. It all just didn't seem real, even as I watched my belly grow and I felt my little boy kick inside me; it just felt too good to be true. It was these feelings that stopped me from truly enjoying my pregnancy. In many ways, I felt that if I did relax and maybe allow myself to believe that this might all work out, that I would somehow jinx our good luck.

Even though I was open about my pregnancy in general, I still felt hesitant about buying actual baby products (clothes, toys, even nursery furnishings). These feelings went way past my first trimester, and each time I contemplated making a purchase, I found myself hesitating, and even wondering whom I could give the item to if things didn't work out. This mindset must sound incredibly insane, and at times I had to almost shake myself and allow myself to enjoy some of those small milestones of my pregnancy as it progressed.

When I was in Australia and just over fifteen weeks pregnant, my mother asked if she could buy a few small items of clothing for our baby. It was her gift as Nana, and given our distance I found myself giving in to this lovely gesture of hers. For my mum, this was an important event for her – her daughter was having a baby, and I really wanted to enjoy the entire experience. Yet, as we browsed the shops, I still found myself hesitating as I touched the small items of clothing. It all felt surreal, and it wasn't until that moment that I even allowed myself in the baby aisles. Don't get me wrong, I loved the experience – shopping with my mum – but there was also a part of me wondering how I would cope if I had to find a way to give these sweet and dinky little outfits away. I felt that at fifteen weeks I was being too presumptuous about the pregnancy with still twenty-five weeks to go.

This one shopping venture didn't make me any more comfortable in my views. When we returned from Australia I didn't buy anything else, not for a long while. That hesitation lingered for many more weeks, and rightly so after some of the hiccups we faced on our way home from Australia. To be honest, I don't think that anxiety ever really disappeared. For me, it was purely self-protection.

It was just after we reached twenty weeks that my husband suggested starting the nursery. I was nervous. However, I knew we needed to get going or we could end up with him sleeping in a cupboard drawer. So I gave in, and we started decorating the small room we had agreed to allocate to our baby boy. It was a step forward, and each morning as I passed by that small room, I found myself smiling with the hope of what was to come. It was a good start to a positive future for us as parents.

Once the nursery was done, it was as though I gave myself permission to take some further steps. Another milestone for me was actually showing off my bump. Until about twenty or so weeks, I found myself wearing loose clothing, concealing my growing belly in the hope of avoiding comments from strangers or even colleagues from work. Whilst I wasn't ashamed of my pregnancy, I was still anxious about the comments and questions that followed from those who weren't as aware of my history. Those who might assume that it had all been smooth sailing and that my pregnancy was a dream experience. However, as my belly grew it became more difficult to hide it, and finally I took the plunge to wear actual maternity clothing, allowing my bump to take a more obvious form in my attire.

It didn't take long before people commented, asking the standard and expected questions such as, when I was due, what the gender might be, or even names. Strangely, I found that with each new comment, my comfort level started to increase. I was no longer talking about loss or infertility; I was now able to talk about our future as parents. I could talk about being a 'mum'! Seeing my bump, feeling him move, and talking about what would happen when our baby was born helped me to become excited about the pregnancy. I liked it when people complimented me on my growing round bump, and I shrugged off the stories of sleepless nights and feeding habits (they were a given after all). I focused on the stories of unconditional love, newborn baby smells and that first moment when we would finally meet our little boy. For the first time in this pregnancy I found myself really beginning to picture our little baby, dreaming about that moment when I would get to hold him in my arms, and those first moments after his birth when it would be the three of us: me, my husband and our son! Those thoughts gave me goose bumps and my heart would beat fast with pure joy and excitement.

Listening for the Rain

Many people warned me that we would be sleep deprived once our baby arrived. I was told to get lots of sleep now and enjoy the quiet time. Well that advice is all well and good, but as the weeks progressed I found myself over-thinking everything, and most of that happened late at night or in the very early hours of the morning. I'm sure no one is surprised by this admission, but as my comfort levels decreased, I found it harder to sleep at night, and as I tossed and turned I would wake myself up as I waited to feel my baby move inside my belly. I was definitely happiest and most at ease when I could feel him, but the vicious cycle here is that I would lie awake smiling to myself as he wriggled about and kicked me. Then as everything went quiet (he was probably sleeping), I would keep myself awake waiting for him to move again.

Then there was the heartburn, his hiccups, or the aches in my legs and back as I struggled to get myself into the right position to relax and fall asleep. On average, I was getting maybe four hours sleep a night. Surely, that's not sustainable?

On the nights when I really struggled, I found myself walking through the house in the dark, throughout the most unsociable of hours. I didn't want to wake my husband with my constant tossing in bed, and I couldn't just lie next to him. Most nights I found myself wide awake and getting up and out of bed was the only solution. I'd sometimes stand in the nursery and try to imagine a baby bringing the newly decorated room to life. Other times, I would sit in our study and write or just fool around on social media. Then the morning would come and I'd be so tired I could barely get myself to work. You would think that I could then get a full night's sleep that following night? Wrong. The cycle would start again.

I was starting to get anxious about the fact that I wasn't sleeping well. Was this good for the baby? What could I do to relax myself? I tried lavender-filled baths before bedtime and warm soothing teas to calm my body and my senses. I switched off all my electrical devices so that I wasn't tempted to pick them up as I lay awake in frustration and I refused to watch television before I slept, so that I wouldn't stimulate my senses. On top of this, there was the constant need to pee. I don't mean just a few times a night; I'm talking hourly trips to the bathroom, sometimes even more! There were nights where I thought it would be more productive to bring my pillow to the bathroom!

After all of this, and just as I would start to drift off to sleep, the little monkey inside my belly would start doing somersaults. Naturally, I couldn't get upset as I felt his movements; instead I would lie there revelling in his little kicks and punches, or his hiccups, placing my hand over the spots where I could feel him as he battered my ribs or lower belly. My heart was tied to this little menace, and I was in awe of the entire experience. Each night, this same pattern continued, but at the same time I was a glutton to the high of feeling my baby moving inside me, and sleep eluded me.

I started to feel myself really struggling as the weeks progressed. I was constantly tired and I must have looked like the walking dead to my work colleagues. Whilst I knew I couldn't sustain this pattern, especially working full-time in a busy role, I didn't know how to reverse the cycle. I had planned to have two weeks' maternity leave before baby arrived, but I still had weeks to go before I finished work.

"Perhaps this is my body's way of preparing me for the little sleep we will have when he arrives..." I joked to my husband one night as my body fell into bed with the heaviness of sleep. I knew I was exhausted but I had little hope that I would actually have a full night's sleep regardless.

"I think you need to just go with it. You're fighting your body and getting far too anxious about not sleeping. The worry is over. We are having our baby. He will be here before we both know it!"

He was right, too. I could keep fretting over not sleeping or I could just give into the fact that I was big, uncomfortable and probably not going to sleep well through the night for the next several weeks.

The best part of it all was that big bright light at the end of this tunnel, and it was lit with millions of different beautiful colours. That rainbow of ours was soon to arrive and I couldn't resent any part of this experience one little bit. It was all part of our journey. In the grand scheme of things, the sleep deprivation was not worth the worry.

In a strange way, once I gave myself permission not to sleep and to just go with the flow, I did actually start to sleep a little better. I certainly didn't ever get a full night's rest, but I felt more relaxed throughout the night. On the nights where I really struggled, I decided to make productive use of the quiet time. I wrote entries into my journal and I worked on personal projects that I might not have had time to do during the day. I would, at times, just sit quietly in the dark with my hands on my belly feeling the little baby boy in there move and kick about, and I'd envision our future together, as a family. With each week we were a step closer to meeting him, and the anticipation was growing immensely.

As the Storm Clears

Everyone kept telling me that the third trimester would go so quickly. I really hoped that it would. I was literally busting to meet my little man, and there have been times where I've felt as though the weeks have crawled by during this pregnancy. Suddenly, however, I realised that I'm well into the home stretch and that there were only a handful of weeks to go before my planned C-section date.

It did feel strange to say that I knew exactly the date and almost the time that my son would be born. Some might have said it takes away some of the mystery and surprise during those final stages of the pregnancy. For me, however, it helped to know that I would have everything in place to ensure the safe delivery of my baby. I've had too many obstacles on this road to even contemplate taking a risk at this late stage. I had been told that I may have adhesions, and I was therefore at risk of haemorrhaging or worse. My baby was also measuring big, and there were question marks over whether I could have a natural delivery with my history. The professional guidance from my consultant was to consider a planned C-section, and I wasn't going to challenge her. Doctor knows best!

In many ways, I was quite content with this approach. Yes, it takes the spontaneity away from the process of labour, but for me, it also means that the entire process will be controlled, monitored and as risk-free as possible given my history. My ultimate goal was to hold that baby boy in my arms. How I got there in the end was of no concern to me. As long as he was safe and healthy, I really didn't care.

So once the date was set, I was literally counting down the weeks and days until the morning we would pack our bags and head to hospital. It was all a very civilised approach. With a set date and time for our C-section, we knew our baby's birthday, and we could plan family and visits around the event. My husband could even ensure his work had exact dates of his paternity leave. It was all planned for week thirty-nine of our pregnancy (exactly one week before my actual due date). It was exciting!

Yet suddenly I felt a senseless last minute panic starting to set in.

"I'm not sure how to be an actual mother!" I said to my husband one evening as we ate dinner.

"Huh?" he said, looking at me confused, unsure of how he should respond. I'm sure he must have thought my outburst quite crazy, given we'd strived to become parents for so long now.

I tried to explain. "Well... we are going to be parents in a few weeks. I really don't know how to be a mum. What if I'm terrible?"

I was searching for reassurance. I needed to know we would be okay. I had wanted this for so long, and yet now it was all becoming far too real. I was going to become a mum! A mum! The word itself suddenly threw a mountain of responsibility on me. I needed to ensure he fed well and he was clean, healthy, devoid of any infections. What if I couldn't make him happy? What if he got sick? Did I know what to do? As the questions mounted in my mind, I felt a sudden pressure rising.

I know my husband saw the panic in my eyes, and in his calm and always sensible manner, he placed his hand on my arm. "We will be fine! We have this."

"Do we?" I asked again, seeking more reassurance.

He simply nodded. His words didn't totally appease the concern but I knew we were in this together. We did have this. "We might not do it all right, but we will learn." He looked me in the eyes waiting for me to respond. "Yes?" he asked, his words pushing me to give myself the confidence boost I needed.

"Yes," I nodded hesitantly.

"You know how to do this. I've seen you with your nephews. You are meant to be a mum!"

I smiled at his words. He knew me too well. I felt my chest release from the fear constraining me and I relaxed as his hand stroked my arm. We did have this! We were meant to be parents and this was our time!

A Dark Cloud

Being pregnant and knowing that I am nurturing and growing a human being is an absolutely unreal concept. As I reached the final weeks of my pregnancy with just five weeks left until my caesarean section, I was still feeling surreal about the entire pregnancy. It was as though I had to keep reinforcing the fact that I was going to have my baby. I was finally going to get to hold my little baby boy in my arms. I still couldn't believe it was actually happening for me. In fact, there was still a dark part of me that remained worried it would all go wrong.

I had to continually stop myself from thinking that way. We had come too far. Perhaps it was the struggles and the early losses, but there was nothing now standing in my way. So why couldn't I get these constant fears to just disappear? I kept telling myself I was being paranoid, but regardless, it was always there. I had to keep focusing on the fact that we had made it this far, that we were the fortunate couple – one of the rare couples who had made it through their fertility challenges. Trust me, I truly do consider myself fortunate to be here, despite the many hiccups we've faced. Even with those few bumps that we have endured throughout the pregnancy, I knew in my heart we were lucky. I kept telling myself that perhaps it has been some strange way of testing my will power and my longed-for desire to become a mother. Whatever the case, I am almost there and I am truly grateful. It didn't stop me, however, from wishing that those last few weeks would just speed up. I wanted nothing more but to be assured of my son's safe delivery!

Just when I thought we couldn't have faced anymore, another obstacle fell in my path. At thirty-five weeks pregnant, I'll admit that my anxiety levels have been truly tested. As I write this chapter in the very early hours of the morning whilst everyone else is asleep and the night sky is clear, I contemplate on the events of the past week. Yes, my mind is running overtime, and I feel I'm truly being tested. Anyone who knows me well understands my determination and intense desire to achieve what I set out for; so above everything I know I will continue to remain strong. I have to. It's not just me anymore – there is a little person who will be here soon, and he needs me more than ever.

However, its been just over twenty-four hours and I am sure I haven't felt my baby move. It is one of those things. I wasn't sure if I was imagining it, whether I should be worried or whether I was just over-thinking things once again. The thing is, once I had it in my head that he wasn't moving, it was all I could think about. The weather had grown very warm, and a part of me was conscious that perhaps he could be running out of space in my belly. Nonetheless, I had a continuing nagging doubt clouding over me. It was only earlier in the year when a good friend of mine had reduced movement and if it weren't for her asking her midwife, her beautiful girl would not be with us today. She was rushed to hospital and her baby was born at thirty-one weeks. Doctors told my friend that had they waited a few more hours, it would have been a very different scenario for that baby's future. Stories like that send shivers down my spine and I kept telling myself, I've come too far to take any risks!

Sitting up in the early hours of the morning, I waited for some kind of movement or sign that things were okay. I drank a lot of cold water, and lay very still for long periods throughout the next morning. Over the past weeks, I had grown to know my baby's pattern, and I knew that there was a difference over the past twenty-four hours. My consultant had advised me to call if there were *any* changes in his movements. Again, I didn't want to over-react or cause a fuss, but it was really starting to play on my mind now. I continued to monitor for the next twelve hours. I couldn't think of anything else. I felt like I was just lying in wait for something significant to happen inside my belly to reassure me.

Despite a few lazy rolls, I knew that the movement I was feeling was different. I called the hospital, and they requested that I come in immediately for monitoring. I felt reassured by the nurse on the phone who told me that I was doing the right thing by coming in to be checked.

It was a Saturday evening, and my husband and I arrived at the hospital at around eight. I still felt silly, but the nursing staff reassured me that it was better to be safe than sorry. The monitoring took about an hour, and we heard his healthy heartbeat and there were a few sluggish movements recorded. I was told that our baby was fine from all their monitoring, but that the decrease in movement could be dehydration, the heat, or perhaps his size. The doctor on call suggested a follow up scan on the following Monday.

I was comforted by the hospital, its staff, and their responsiveness to my situation. I still felt a little silly and wondered if it was perhaps my anxious mind playing tricks on me. However, regardless of anything, I just couldn't risk it. We had come too far to even test the odds at this stage. When Monday came, our scan showed that our baby's growth had increased a lot, and he was measuring over the ninety-fifth percentile. At the time, I was almost thirty-six weeks and he was weighing well over six pounds. I was referred to undergo a second gestational diabetes test, despite my negative test at twenty-six weeks. It was that, or he was just a very big baby. Either way, it was another worry to add to my growing list.

My test did come back positive this time, and given my family history with diabetes I guess it wasn't a huge surprise that I had gestational diabetes. I hadn't been consuming a lot of sugars, but my body had become less able to process them – even a spoonful of sugar in my morning tea was creating sugar highs that neither I or my baby could handle. A strict diet was given to me, and daily testing of my blood sugars was prescribed. It wasn't a huge obstacle but it was another hiccup on this road. With just three weeks to go, I was so anxious to meet my little boy, and I wasn't sure if I could face any more set backs. Well, I was wrong!

When I received an urgent call from my mum in Australia with some difficult news, I really did question how much more I could take. My father had been rushed to hospital once more. Suddenly, for some reason, his legs stopped working. He couldn't stand, and he had fallen and couldn't get back up. My dad is a big man and my mum wasn't able to assist him; she couldn't even lift him from the ground to support his weight. An ambulance was called and he was taken straight to the local hospital for tests. I was on the phone to my mum at regular intervals, and as the situation progressed, it was clear that his legs were not the only issue. Once he was admitted to hospital, it was clear that my father was also experiencing bouts of paranoia and becoming somewhat delusional. The medical staff advised that this was either the cancer progressing, or perhaps he had suffered another stroke. Either way, it didn't seem promising.

I felt helpless. I was so far away, and all I wanted was to see my dad. He had held on this far, but I had to wonder how much more strength he had in him to fight. I wasn't even able to fly there to support my mum and my brother. I was thirty-six weeks pregnant and growing by the day; I was barely able to make it to the local shops.

My dad's cancer was becoming all too real, and it became clear that he might not be able to go home again. He may have to go into full time care. His condition was certainly worsening, and whilst he still had lucid moments, my mum explained that he was losing time, places, forgetting names and sometimes reverting to experiences within his past. How must he feel? Without sitting in front of him, I could only imagine how scared he must have been. It felt so cruel, and whilst I wanted him to fight this disease, most of all, I didn't want him to suffer. By all accounts, he was struggling with the hospital and couldn't understand why he was there.

However, he was no longer fit enough to be at home; he needed full-time medical care.

    Selfishly, I wanted to see him one last time. I was hoping I could fly home a few months after the birth of our son, and introduce him to his grandson. I knew I couldn't keep my dad forever, but he had come this far, and I just needed him to hang on for a few more months. I wanted that one more moment with him. I wanted him to see me as a mum, as I knew he had been so excited about this pregnancy. I wondered now how likely that would be. Perhaps I was asking too much, but I couldn't help but hope that this one last wish would fall in my favour.

The Clear Night Sky

I'm sure I was becoming a pest, but each day I phoned my mum for an update on Dad's condition. It was difficult for Mum, as she played the liaison between the hospital staff, consultants, family and my dad, and I knew that the waiting was beginning to wear on her. By all accounts, my dad wasn't himself. He had become agitated about being in the hospital, and the man who was always called a 'gentle giant' seemed to be losing his temper at the most frivolous of things. It was most certainly the cancer or the radiation treatment he had undergone affecting his brain and his reactions. He was scared and he felt isolated being in the hospital and unable to go home. It was devastating to be just a bystander to it all.

My mum tells me that he still knows that I am pregnant, and that he is eagerly waiting on this baby boy to be born. I was so reassured to hear this. Perhaps it is the anticipation that is keeping him fighting. If anything, it has made me more determined to get through these last through weeks with positivity and determination. My own anxieties are nothing compared to what my dad is going through right now.

It would be at least a few months before I could fly to Australia, but I planned to bombard him with photos and videos of his latest grandson. It was my hope that this would be the incentive for him to fight long enough so that I could plan a trip home within the first three months of my son's birth. At this stage, we could only take one day at a time.

As I reached my thirty-seventh week, I had a consultant appointment to discuss the birth and any other final matters on this pregnancy. It was as though fate was playing its cards in my favour as I sat down with the consultant and his assistant. As he went through my file and everything I've been through, he made the suggestion that we bring the caesarean forward one week. His reasoning was mainly due to the size of our baby, but also the episode of reduced movement and my risk of going into labour naturally. I'll admit I was a little thrown as the date he gave me was six days away. I would be having a baby in less than a week.

I'm sure I felt my heart stop at that moment with the reality of what that meant. I was going to have a baby! Our baby! Our Rainbow Baby! It was all becoming so real.

I know many women would protest at bringing their labour early, but for me, it was the news I needed. The consultant assured me that there was very limited risk to bringing forward our delivery date, and that I was ready to have our baby. I wasn't prepared to risk going into a natural labour early, and when I told my dad he was ecstatic. Our baby's due date was in arm's reach and it was exciting. All this time, all those struggles and obstacles, and finally we would have our beautiful baby to hold.

As the days progressed towards our scheduled delivery date, my mum gave me some good news. Dad had turned a corner. His doctor thought that perhaps it was a small stroke, and that it had caused some swelling on the brain. However, he was reverting to his old self, and becoming much more positive, which was wonderful to hear. It felt as though the dark cloud looming over us was finally clearing. As the days progressed, I felt more confident that I would see my dad in person again and he would be able to meet his baby grandson.

Our rainbow was starting to appear and there were no clouds in sight to take it away from us now!

I Can See a Rainbow

I could barely sleep all night with the anticipation. We had our alarms set for six in the morning, as we had to be at the hospital by seven-thirty. It wasn't as if I needed an alarm however, it wasn't even a possibility that I would sleep through our required departure time. I was ready for this. I had waited for more than nine months; I'd been waiting for this moment for almost five years now!

As we walked into the hospital, it was all very civilised. We had the bag packed, but unlike the standard labour I'd envisioned, there was no panic, urgency or pain. We walked up to reception and we were shown to a small hospital bed, where I was told to dress, and be ready to be called. It was strange.

As we sat waiting, we spoke of trivial matters. It was all a little surreal for both of us. I'd been in hospital plenty of times before waiting for a 'procedure', but this was different. This wasn't just a 'procedure'; this was the birth of our first-born child. This was what we had been striving for over the past four years. It was a momentous occasion, and I just cannot describe the feeling as we sat there ready to be called, waiting for the moment where we would get to meet our son.

Like most hospitals, they were running late, and we were told that an emergency procedure meant that the schedule was running behind time. It wasn't a surprise, and there was certainly no urgency for us at this point of time. Regardless, my heart seemed to pulse erratically each time the door opened to the waiting room and the anticipation was making my head fuzzy. It was becoming all so real.

Finally, two hours after our scheduled 'procedure' time, a nurse walked in. "Are you ready?" she asked.

I could only nod and I followed her, grabbing my husband's hand to stay close by me. Was I ready? Of course I was, but still a lump in my throat prevented me from even being able to speak.

As we entered a small sterile hall, my husband was veered off to get into scrubs, and I was led into a large room with a small bed in the very middle.

"Are you ready to have your baby?" the nurse asked me as she led me towards the small bed.

Tears started to fall from my eyes. It was overwhelming. I looked around and there were doctors and nurses preparing themselves and their equipment. They were doing all of this for my son and me. I really didn't know what to expect from the C-section, and all I could think of was that soon I would hold my son. Soon I would finally meet him, see his face, touch him, kiss him, and hold him. The room was stark white and sterile, with blinding lights, but I swear I could see the colours of my rainbow appearing before my glazed eyes.

I won't go into the graphic detail of the C-section, but all I will say was that it was so very straightforward. My husband came into the room once I was prepared and ready to go. He sat beside me throughout the entire procedure. I heard a lot of noises but I didn't feel a thing. Then there was a sound I will never forget.

The wail of our son echoed through the room, and I looked to my husband and he looked at me. We were unable to see anything, as a large curtain separated my husband and I from what the consultants and nurses were doing to birth my son. However, shortly after those ardent cries, the doctor brought our son around the curtain to meet us. He was wonderful!

Small, squirmy, sticky and wonderful – I couldn't believe he was ours. He was quickly cleaned up and we had skin-to-skin time. I was able to finally hold my little man. I'd envisioned this for so long, and we were finally here. I can't explain how full my heart felt; looking at my husband and my son, my world was now complete.

As I look back, and then look at my family now, I will always remember the four angels who passed before. Their brother, our newborn son, will always know that he was part of an incredibly difficult but special journey. As I looked into his small, delicate face, I was in love. Whilst I would never have said this at the time, as I hold my son now, I can say it was all worth the fight, the heartache, the pain, and the uncertainty. The choices I made and the path I followed, led me to this road.

I am now moving into the land of motherhood, and I will do all I can to be the best mother I can be. Perhaps I am a different mother today than what I would have been if I had not experienced the challenges getting to this day. What I can promise is that my son will be cherished, loved and adored – not only by my husband and myself, but also by everyone who knows our journey.

I know that we have been blessed with our miracle. The rainbow we have been searching for is now shining brightly and our storm has well and truly passed.

The Pot of Gold

Thank you for reading my story. It has been a long journey, but I know that many have faced much longer journeys. The struggle with fertility is all too real for many couples. We fought hard for our gorgeous rainbow baby, and we are truly blessed to have him safe and happy in our arms. As I look at my baby, I'm reminded of the might of Mother Nature, and I'm humbled that I've been so fortunate to overcome the issues that caused our earlier losses and our inability to conceive. I'm proud of myself for never giving in, and I will never forget what I've learned from this experience – for the good and bad. It will make me a better mother than I could have ever hoped to be, and gives me the empathy towards other's who are either on their journey or like me, have fought and faced their infertility.

I found my rainbow, and there was a pot of gold at the end of my road. I'm forever rich and I need nothing more. This was all I hoped for – our son is everything I ever wanted.

When my son was only two weeks old, I was able to get him a passport photo and his birth registered, and he had a full passport before he was a month old. As he was born with severe club feet, we requested to start his treatment as early as possible, with his first casts (hip to toe) being set at just over two weeks old. With the treatment schedule to rehabilitate his feet all planned, I was able to book flights back to Australia to fit within his rehabilitation schedule before he reached his third month. In honour of my dad, we gave our son my father's name and when he finally met my dad, his grandpa, he laughed and smiled with delight. It was magical. My dad was in a wonderful place, and he revelled in meeting his newest grandson. My heart could not have been more complete during those moments. My rainbow baby and my father – both amazing fighters and proof that wishes do come true.

Remain hopeful above all things and stay strong, no matter the course.

The End

Thank you for reading my story.

My son, Isaac was born on the 10th August 2016.

He was born with bilateral fixed Talipes feet, with no other issues identified. On publishing this book he is six months old, and completed the major part of his treatment for his feet. He is almost crawling, and certainly showing no developmental delays.

Every day I am thankful for my RAINBOW BABY.

My father continued to fight his cancer, until the 28th May 2017. My son was just over nine months old and we enjoyed regular video calls so that he could watch his grandson's progress. We spoke with him just ten minutes before he left us, and he was still positive until that very last moment. I will always remind my son of his Grandpa and those special moments he had with him.

Finding the Rainbow

Finding the Rainbow was my first memoir, and my first published work. If you haven't read this and would like to, it is a different part of my story. It details the stage of my life where I had made the decision to become a mother, but sadly found out that we would face difficulties in carrying a child to full term.

"...McGrath skillfully weaves the story of their reaching out for the Rainbow Child into a most compelling true-life story. Finding the Rainbow is highly recommended..." ***Readers Favorite, 5 Star Review***

BOOKS BY RACHEL McGRATH

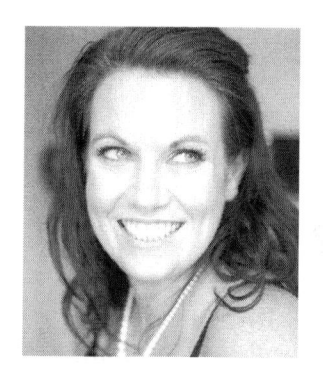

Non-Fiction, Memoir
Finding the Rainbow
Eye of the Storm
Embracing the Storm

Children's Fiction
Mud on your Face
Grimwald's Evil Plan
The Willow and Coco Children's Series

Fiction
Dark & Twisty, A Twisted Anthology
Tortured Minds
Unfinished Chapters (Contributor)

Printed in Great Britain
by Amazon